Can't S
Won't ?

Linda Louisa Dell

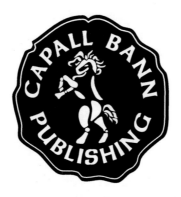

www.capallbann.co.uk

Can't Sleep, Won't Sleep

Cover design by Paul Mason
Author photograph on back cover by Paul Higgins
Cover sketch idea by Jim King
Internal illustrations by Pat Ginter

Published by:

Capall Bann Publishing
Auton Farm
Milverton
Somerset
TA4 1NE

To Amanda

from

Linda Louisa Dell

Dedication

To friends I knew, to friends I know and to friends I have yet
to know.

And the lessons I learned from them all.

Advice to readers

This book aims to give you some of the many reasons for sleep problems and to list some of the many remedies, therapies and techniques that can help you to re-train your sleep patterns to your very individual needs.

This book is not intended as guidance for the treatment of serious health problems and I would always advise you to refer to your doctor if you have any serious health worries.

You should also always inform your doctor of any complementary medicines and remedies you are taking in particular if you are taking any prescribed medications.

March 2005

Men who are unhappy, like men who sleep badly,
are always proud of the fact.
The conquest of happiness, Bertrand Russell

Contents page

Foreword

Insomnia

According to the British Medical Association, one in three adults may suffer from insomnia at some time in their lives. Fortunately for most people this is a temporary inconvenience, though often a rather debilitating one. Unfortunately, there are many who lose the battle with Morpheus - the god of sleep - nightly.

Writing as one who has experienced a lifetime of sleepless nights, I feel very pleased that a book like this is available to give hope to my fellow insomniacs and myself. We all know that whilst one remedy may work for one individual, it has absolutely no effect on another. That is why this is a great little book: it offers so many different ways of combating this nocturnal nuisance. What is more important is that the remedies are natural and dispense with reliance on drugs (unless its what the doctor orders of course). If anyone is on prescription drugs of course, its just as well to always let the doctor know if other remedies are sought for any condition, even if that remedy is naturally derived.

Perhaps the most debilitating aspect of insomnia is the difficulty in coping with life next day. Fatigue, irritability and a general lack of joy, are but some of the consequences of a sleepless night. There are of course, many different causes for insomnia. Some are temporary, as we know; other reasons may derive from an innate predisposition perhaps. But its true to say of course, that the amount needed to rest one's weary head differs from person to person. Whilst it's often said that we need about eight hours per night that might be just too much for some people.

Our nocturnal habits differ in the way we sleep, or not as the case may be. Some lie there for hours praying for that unconscious state, whilst others fall asleep at the drop of a hat only to wake in the middle of the night, quite alert, and stay that way until morning. Or until it's time to get up and then the heavy cloak of sleep begins to overtake them, just when it's too late.

The causes of insomnia are many and these have been outlined in detail in this book. No doubt the insomniac will be familiar with his/her particular case and hopefully find themselves considering a new way of dealing with the old demon.

This is a wonderful book and really needs no introduction. It covers just about everything any insomniac can think of, and probably more. It's a delight to read from cover to cover, or just to dip into now and again, perhaps on one of those sleepless nights.

Wanda Sellar
February 2004
Holistic Writer and author of
The Directory of Essential Oils publisher C.W. Daniel & Co. Ltd
Frankincense & Myrrh (with Martin Watt) publisher C.W. Daniel & Co.Ltd
'*The Consultation Chart*, pub: Wessex Astrologer

Introduction

It is estimated that only about one in five of us sleeps well with little effort, the rest need to work at it. I hope that this book will help you to improve the quality of your sleep in an easy, effective and natural way. It will also help you get more from your sleep, perhaps in ways that you cannot now imagine, by making you a more contented person who is more satisfied with life and is easier to get along with. As adults in the modern world, we face many challenges and responsibilities, stress and anxiety at work, demands from; the care of children, shift work, commuting and international travel take their toll, making good quality sleep more important, but unfortunately more difficult than ever to achieve. You may have picked up this book because you, or someone you know, have insomnia or other sleep-related problems, such as snoring or restless leg syndrome, and the quality of your life is being affected. You may already have tried prescribed medications, and found that they are effective for a short while, and then the problem slowly returns.

All too often, sleep problems are attributed to stress, hormones, being over weight, having young children or working unsociable hours. These things are all relevant, and can contribute to insomnia. Many of these preconditions can be overcome with positive thinking and professional help. Poor sleep causes sleepiness during the day, which can lead to accidents, poor performance at work and decreased job satisfaction, bad moods and inadequate social skills. Depleted sleep affects our general health and ability to thrive, the heart, brain and digestive system, resistance to illness; regulation of the natural aging process and our relationships can also suffer.

The first part of this book covers what sleep is and why we need it, what insomnia is, and why we dream. The second part gives a break down of the many possible causes and contributory ailments for sleep problems and insomnia. The third part gives a breakdown of the many remedies, techniques and complementary therapies available that can help to ease and combat insomnia and sleep problems. The 4th part will tell you how to choose a therapist and give you some checklists and information about keeping a sleep diary. You can learn to sleep and dream peacefully, and waking up refreshed and energized will soon become normal for you.

If you remember the joy and peace of restful sleep you will understand why it is worth devoting some time and effort to get a better nights sleep.

PART ONE

Chapter 1

What is Insomnia?

Insomnia is the inability to fall asleep and stay asleep, and many people will tell you that they have experienced it at some time in their lives. If it is only a problem occasionally, you can usually identify the cause and do something about it – noise or light pollution, too much coffee close to bedtime, or some other external cause. But for those who have to deal regularly with insomnia, it interferes dramatically on their daily lives.

There are three types of insomnia: insomnia can be classified as transient (short term), intermittent (on and off), and chronic (constant). Insomnia lasting from a single night to a few days is referred to as transient. If episodes of transient insomnia occur frequently, the insomnia is said to be intermittent. Insomnia is considered to be chronic if it occurs on most nights and lasts a month or more. According to research in Pharmacy magazine: Nine percent of sufferers say they have had an accident because of sleepiness and it has cost the country an estimated £11 million in lost production. Many millions of people in the UK suffer from chronic insomnia, defined as poor sleep every night or most nights, and even more Americans also complain of chronic insomnia. One in three people are likely to have some form of insomnia at some time in their lives, and in England and Wales doctors write out more than twenty million prescriptions for sleeping pills each year. The annual drugs bill for prescribed sleeping pills is £58 million and many people take them for years on end – often with problems of withdrawal and side effects, which can include anxiety and restlessness. The number of hour's sleep a person needs or how long it takes to fall asleep does not define insomnia. Individuals vary normally in their need for, and satisfaction from sleep. However, when an individual cannot get to sleep, and stay asleep, for the duration that they need, then they are suffering from insomnia.

Who is Likely to Experience Insomnia?
Women seem to be more prone to insomnia than men, as are the elderly of both sexes, the terminally ill, those in chronic pain and individuals with a history of depression.

Conditions such as stress, anxiety, certain medical problems, or the use of certain medications, together with the above circumstances, mean that insomnia is much more likely. Indeed, some experts say that personality will play a part in your sleep needs, it is sometimes said that ambitious, driven people need less sleep than more relaxed, contented individuals who are able to sleep longer. The reasons for insomnia are not always clear-cut, and insomniacs do not generally fall into any set social, economic or educational groups.

What Causes Transient and Intermittent Insomnia?
Transient and intermittent insomnia generally occur in people who are temporarily experiencing one or more of the following: stress, environmental noise pollution, extremes of temperatures, changes in the surrounding environment such as; moving from a quiet area to a noisy town center, sleep/wake schedule problems, such as those caused by shift

work, jet lag or a new baby. These temporary disturbances can be rectified with time and proper management, techniques for which are described in the following chapters.

What Causes Chronic Insomnia?

Chronic insomnia is more complex and often results from a combination of factors, including physical or mental disorders - one of the most common causes of chronic insomnia is depression. Other causes include arthritis, kidney disease, heart problems, asthma, sleep apnoea, narcolepsy, restless legs syndrome, Parkinson's disease, hyperthyroidism and chronic stress.. However, chronic insomnia may also be due to behavioural factors, including the misuse of caffeine, alcohol, or other substances.

What is the Purpose of Sleep?

On average, human beings spend a third of their lives in sleep, yet scientists do not yet know precisely what sleep accomplishes. It is assumed to serve some restorative function, but just how sleep refreshes us is unclear. Whatever the function of sleep, the need for it is undeniable as any insomniac will testify. A certain amount of regeneration takes place while we sleep, dead and dying cells in our bodies are replaced at a faster pace while we are asleep than when we are awake. Throughout our sleep certain growth hormones reach their peak activity and many enzyme reactions increase. Sleep is also seen as a means of maintaining our mental health. It is a period during which we can 'withdraw' from the world and sort through the events of the day. Through our dreams we are continually able to deal with and store new information and feelings. Furthermore, many researchers view our need for sleep as a behavioural pattern inherited from our primitive ancestors. Their survival depended, in part, on their avoiding the dangers of the dark night. Sleeping away the night in the security of the cave successfully accomplished this. This pattern is repeated in the animal kingdom. Animals that are seldom attacked sleep for much longer and more deeply than those which are prey, and which need to be more vigilant against attack. Such as rabbits whom shelter in their burrows during the dark night hours, whereas the lion can slumber away the day without fear of attack. One thing that is sure is that sleep is not a passive state. Electroencephalography, the study of electrical impulses from the cerebral cortex, shows that the human brain is anything but inactive while you are sleeping. Sleep-deprivation experiments reveal that when human beings are compelled to stay awake, they begin to function less capably than usual after only 24 hours. After about ten sleepless days, they have trouble carrying out mental and physical tasks, and their judgment and memory deteriorate. If they're kept awake long enough they may hallucinate and show other signs of mental disturbance. A recent study found that sleep deprived surgeons make around 20 per cent more errors and are 14 per cent slower than colleagues who have had some rest. Enforced sleeplessness also tends to break down willpower and to make people less vigilant and more suggestible. That is why sleep deprivation has often been imposed by unscrupulous police officers trying to extract confessions, by military interrogators hoping to gain information from wartime prisoners, and by political brain washers seeking to win converts to their way of thinking.

What is Sleep?

Hypnology is the name for the science of the phenomena of sleep, there are now sleep centres at many hospitals and the study of sleep problems are becoming more prominent within the medical profession. The brain is not inactive during sleep but sleep is usually defined as a time when an animal stops responding to its surroundings in any active outward appearance. Sleep is a normal, regular state of rest for any animal organism, in contrast to the waking state; sleep is distinguished by a low level of physiological functions; such as blood pressure, breathing, and the rate of heartbeat. Most animals close their eyes, and many adopt a specific posture; dogs and cats curl up, bats hang upside down, and other animals (cows, horses) can sleep standing up. Birds sleep for only seconds or minutes at a time and some birds can sleep while flying or swimming. Sleep experts were amazed to learn that many marine mammals (such as dolphins) and almost all birds can sleep with only one side of the brain at a time, while the other side remains awake. This is known as 'unihemispheric sleep'. This way of sleeping is clearly sensible for a mammal that breathes air but lives underwater; to be completely asleep and unable to swim to the surface for air would mean drowning. For birds the advantage of unihemipheric sleep is that they can sleep and look out for predators simultaneously. Humans may have this ability to sleep with only part of the brain at a time, many a mother will state that they were fast asleep but awoke instantly that their child or baby cried, but certainly not to the same degree as dolphins and whales.

Does Everyone Need Eight Hours of Sleep a Night?

People need enough sleep to make them wake refreshed. That may mean no more than three/four hours a night for a very few mortal beings, Margaret Thatcher is said to only sleep four hours per night. Leonardo da Vinci tried a different approach to sleep, rather than cutting down his main sleep period, he slept for twenty minutes every two hours, which adds up to about four hours in every day. Five or six hours are usual for many adults, seven or eight for most is about right, and in some cases as many as nine hours or more may be needed. A newborn baby will require 16-18 hours of sleep in a 24 hour period, reducing to 14-15 hours by age one, 10-12 by age four, and less than 10 by age ten. Sleep needs further reduce as adolescence progresses although some teenagers

The Brain and Spinal cord

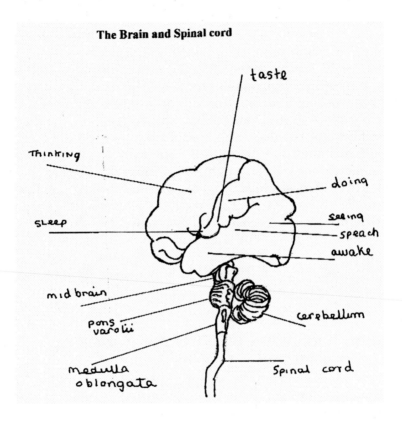

taste

Thinking

doing

sleep

seeing
speach
awake

mid brain

pons
varolii

cerebellum

medulla
oblongata

spinal cord

can sleep for 10-12 hours, and this could be that sleep is needed for the rapid growth needed in puberty. The length of average sleep stabilizes at about 7-8 hours in adulthood for most people, it is accepted that two thirds of the adult population sleep for an average seven and a half hours a night. The elderly tend to lose their capacity for prolonged sleep but will often doze during the daytime. (see chart pg..)The true measure of how much sleep you require is how rested you feel when you wake up, if you wake refreshed after only five hours, and are not tired and restless during the day, then five hours sleep is enough for you.

How The Brain Works When You Sleep?

Disturbed sleep can be either neuronic (based on neurons) or neurotic (based on mental state). Neuronic theories include all hormone and other biological influences on sleep.

The sleep awake and clock centers interact with the higher center in the brain and inevitably must interact with the mind. Experts argue that the pattern of nerve cell (neuron) firing is a mental state. Neurons are located in the brain stem in the lower part of the brain that connects the spinal cord with the brain. This is also the area that contains parts of the "awake" center. A tremendous amount of knowledge has been accumulated about the central and peripheral mechanisms controlling and involving sleep. Basically, certain areas in the brain stem, the most fundamental part of the brain, and the part that controls such basic functions as breathing and heart rate, are involved in the control of the sleep stages. Several brain chemicals called biogenic amines are involved called; dopamine, noradrenaline, serotonin, these act as transmitters regulating brain cells.

The brain waves constantly change during the sleep cycle and go in waves of lighter and deeper sleep throughout the night. The brain, with its intricate covering of grey matter, the cortex, looks something like a walnut. (see chart page 10) It is considered that the two halves or hemispheres of the brain reflect our dual nature. The left hemisphere tends to deal with logical thinking, analysis, mathematics, and linear and verbal concepts. The right hemisphere tends to deal with creative thinking, artistic, aesthetic, spatial, non-linear and intuitive matters. People are sometimes described as 'right' or 'left' brained, meaning that they seem to have such an emphasis to their personality.

The two hemispheres are symmetrical, and both have a sensory, motor, visual and auditory area. For the most part however, functions on the right side of the body are controlled by the left hemisphere and vice versa. This is because the major motor nerves cross over as they leave the brain. Each hemisphere is divided into four lobes: frontal, parietal, occipital and temporal. What is necessary is to turn off the right side of the brain, the active, thinking and creative part. Apparently, on the point of sleep, the right cerebral hemisphere is freed from its usual domination by the left side of the brain allowing rest and relaxation to take place. The normally dominant left hemisphere tends to control; language, writing, calculation, science and logic, the right hemisphere is more concerned with spatial construction and pattern sense. So mundane tasks like ironing, cleaning your shoes are ideal jobs for just before bed, juggling also stimulates the right side of the brain, so juggling can help you sleep.

Dreaming
Some psychologists believe sleep to be a time when suppressed emotional issues are dealt with through dreams. We are able to throw out useless information and deal with emotions such as anger and frustration, so that these emotions are not repressed to the point where they can become damaging. When sleep is denied, or we don't go into

REM sleep, these feelings and frustrations can boil over into our every day lives, by not allowing us to renew ourselves and prepare our minds for the new day. (see chapter 11 sleep-walking, violence or other activity in sleep) Psychosomatic illness (physical illness with a psychological origin) is said to account for many disorders such as high blood pressure, headaches, and stomach ulcers.

Dealing with emotional issues through dreams may help to prevent suppressed feelings such as anger, grief, and envy from manifesting as physical symptoms. Record your dreams, learn from them, and let them be a time of release. Dreams are part of the process of human development, and whether the individual notices it or not, dreams will be a contributing factor to our efforts to fulfil the whole of our potential, concentrating especially on those parts that we are neglecting and that are therefore threatening growth and development. It is believed by dream experts that we all dream, and that we can train ourselves to remember our dreams. Keep a note pad next to the bed and first thing when you wake up right down anything that you remember. Over a period of time, if you do this every day, you will remember more and more detail from your dreams. (see page 284 for information on keeping a sleep/dream diary) You may find some very relevant pieces of information coming to light through your dreams, revealing how you really feel about certain situations, and your hopes and fears in life. Many ancient cultures saw a connection between dreams and physical and spiritual health, native aboriginal peoples of Australia, and Native Americans still believe in sharing and staging out dreams to release their emotional and creative energy.

We have all had daydreams, or moments of reverie, some people call this reflection, drifting away from the real world, or collecting our thoughts or just resting our minds for a while, this can be an important time allowing us to take stock and gather our thoughts.

Dreams tell us what we need, as well as what we desire, in order to be complete.

Even if you have never remembered a dream in your life, you probably would if a sleep researcher woke you from REM sleep in a laboratory. Some studies have shown that 84 out of 100 people so awakened report a dream in progress. In any case, people seem to have a strong need to dream, and it is possible that dreams are very important to mental health. If a sleep researcher deprives you of dream sleep for a night by waking you every time you fall into REM state, you'll feel tired and irritable the next day, even if you have been allowed eight hours of NREM sleep. And according to trials the first chance you get to sleep undisturbed, you'll dream more or less continuously, as though you had a dream quota to make up.

But Why Should Dreaming Be Essential To Well-being?

Freud would say that dreams let people express forbidden wishes in disguised form. Although the neurologist Richards M. Restak by no means accepts all of Freud's theories, he does believe that some dreams can give us "creative insight" into the mind, our own and other people. Who, Restak asks, "hasn't experienced a prophetic dream, achieved an important insight about another person in a dream, or suddenly discovered a solution to a confusing daytime dilemma in a dream?" Although such dreams can be disturbing, they often shed light on things that are bothering you at a subconscious level.

If the dreams are about choking, drowning, being strangled, or suffocating, investigate whether you have sleep apnoea or nocturnal reflux. If they are about feelings or emotions, ask yourself whether there is some unfinished business in your waking life. Aristotle believed that dreams echoed the state of the body's mental and physical health and could be used to diagnose and treat illness.

14

What Happens When You Sleep And Dream?

There are two principal kinds of sleep, and you normally move from one to the other over approximately 90-minute intervals throughout the night. When you first go to bed, you fall into slow-wave sleep, so named from the fact that brain waves slow down. You gradually drift into a quiet state in which both your temperature and pulse rate drop. This sleep is largely dreamless, and then approximately 90 minutes after you fall asleep, your blood pressure, pulse, and respiration become irregular. The ears are tuned for hearing, and your eyes dart back and forth, as if you were watching a movie. In fact, you are dreaming, this is REM (rapid eye movement) sleep, which is also known as paradoxical sleep because it is unlike the popular idea of sleep as a quiet state. Your brain is as active as when you're awake, and your brain waves resemble those emitted in the daytime. In a normal night, you spend approximately 25 percent of the time in paradoxical sleep.

The main point is that dreaming sleep is an active brain state, and that without specific sleep centers working properly, and wake centers able to shut down, sleep cannot take place.

Circadian Rhythms

Our circadian rhythm runs for one day (24 hours) and is broken down into 90-minute segments called ultradian rhythms. Our normal sleep cycle runs for 90 minutes and is broken down into different lengths of time. Our sleep patterns are set by our lives, jobs, our daily routines and body temperature. As adults it makes sense to time things so that we sleep when it is dark and when our waking activities are limited, work in the morning when our minds and bodies are fresh, and relax in the evening. All of us have a basic biological rhythm of body temperature, highest after midday and lowest at 3 - 5 am.

Under normal circumstances, our sleep is synchronized to this pattern and we find is easier to fall asleep when our body temperature is falling in late evening and easier to wake up when we're warming up in the morning. This rhythm can be thrown out by disturbances to our normal cycle.

The Stages Of Sleep

Sleep is a dynamic process that involves two types of rest: quiet and active. Active sleep is called REM sleep (for Rapid Eye Movement). It is preceded by quiet sleep (NREM), which has four stages. (see chart on next page)

1. This stage lasts between 5 to 10 minutes. All bodily activity starts to slow down, muscles relax, temperature decreases, pulse and respiration become more regular, and one is easily awakened.

2. Bodily movements continue to decrease and one is soundly asleep, yet can be awakened by sounds. At this point, the eyes become unresponsive to stimuli and start to roll back and forth.

3. By this time the body is almost totally relaxed and one is not easily awakened.

4. At this deepest level the muscles are completely at rest and there is little body movement. One awakens very slowly from this stage.

REM sleep, this is the stage where dreams occur, the level of one's nervous and mental activities increases as well as temperature and heart rate. Rapid darting movements of the eyes characterize it. Deep sleep periods (stages three and four) occur more frequently in the early night and REM sleep periods are longer in the later stage of sleep, usually just before natural awakening.

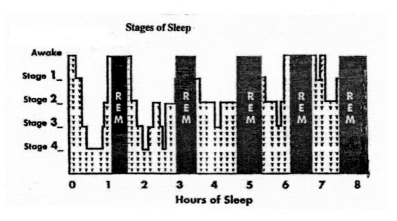

Stages of Sleep

1. When people fall asleep and go to stage 1, NREM to stage 2, stage 3 and finally stage 4. After being asleep for an hour or so people will start moving up from stage 4, NREM to stage 3, then to stage 2 and then to stage 1 again. At this point, approximately ninety minutes after sleep onset, the first REM period of sleep begins.

When you wake up with a jolt from an alarm clock, and you move into your waking state of consciousness, you may have come from a dream state, an out of body state, or a deep sleep state. There are many ways of being woken, when you wake naturally, you are usually at the end of a sleep cycle of about 90 minutes and you come back to the waking state in a few moments. But this is not always the case, if the alarm goes off or you hear a sudden noise or feel a sudden movement, you may experience a number of emotions ranging from irritability to extreme drowsiness. You need to realize that you have left your sleep at a stage, which is not the best time for you, and you may have left something unresolved such as an unfinished dream. Before getting out of bed, take a few moments to gather your thoughts and senses. If you have to set an alarm, give yourself a time allowance to centre yourself, fully wake up and come to properly. If you are in danger of going of to sleep again buy one of those alarm clocks that rings again after 10 minutes.

Sleep Disruptions
A new field of clinical medicine, sleep medicine, is developing, allied to psychiatry and neurology, it deals with all sleep disorders, of which many kinds can now be identified. Sleep problems are usually distributed into three main groups;

• Insomnia: a group of questions generating difficulty in falling asleep or staying asleep.

• Hyper-somnolence: too much sleep, or sleepiness when a person does not want to sleep, such as with narcolepsy

• Episodic nocturnal events, consisting of disorders such as night terrors, nightmares, and sleepwalking or somnambulism.

• Sleep Apnoea

Insomnia and hyper-somnolence are symptoms of sleep problems that may have many different causes. Insomnia is not an illness that can be cured by a sleeping pill. Physicians must determine and treat the insomnia's underlying causes.

Experts estimate that in three quarters of all cases of insomnia the cause is psychological, often after distressing events such as; bereavement or loss of a job, a person may experience sleep difficulties. Many people recover their normal sleep rhythm naturally, but others become frustrated or depressed and develop chronic (long term) insomnia, the most important thing is to realize that you can do something about it. To decide what to do you will need to look at your attitudes, lifestyle and possibly ask yourself a few leading questions. But once you start on a plan of action you will not only improve your sleep pattern, but also start creating for yourself a happier, more satisfying daytime life.

PART TWO

Chapter 2

Contributory Reasons For Insomnia

What Causes Insomnia?

Traffic noise, loud disruptive neighbours, and battered old mattresses are frequently culprits, but among the commonest reasons for chronic insomnia are anxiety and depression. In one study, by Mind, 70 percent of the people who had trouble sleeping suffered from emotional problems. Many physical ailments, especially if they cause breathlessness, fever, or pain, can also make it difficult to sleep, and so can the drugs used to treat asthma, high blood pressure, and other diseases. Abuses of common drugs that affect the brain are often a factor in many cases of insomnia. In others, the trouble may come from working the night shift, going to bed and getting up at irregular hours, or napping in the daytime.

Environmental Factors

The bedroom environment influences our sleep in several ways. The physical environment is an important factor in getting to sleep, and staying asleep. Many people have disrupted sleep because they are too hot, cold, uncomfortable, or are disturbed by noise or light, often without being fully aware of the reason. Your bedroom environment should create a peaceful and tranquil refuge, where you feel safe and secure and able to relax completely into sleep. The psychological environment is as important or even more important than the actual physical, as far as getting to sleep is concerned. (see environmental checklist page 250) One has to feel safe to sleep soundly, if there is the likelihood of being disturbed, if you share a room with someone or generally don't feel safe in your environment you will not relax mentally or physically and sleep is likely to be impaired and disturbed as a result. All the environmental aspects of your bedroom must be considered; heat, light, safety, noise, location of the room, furniture in it and most importantly the bed itself. You want to create a clutter free environment, free from work, computer, television and anything not related to sleep. Electrical equipment creates geopathic stress, which can disrupt normal sleep patterns.

Many sleep disturbances, insomnia, teeth grinding, sleep walking and feeling cold or restless in bed (restless leg syndrome), are all considered signs of geopathic stress. If you have a bedsit, studio flat or have to share your bedroom with an office, try to keep the two areas separate use a screen, curtain or bookcase to divide your sleeping area from your working area. Plants can help, spider plants are a good choice and they are very effective at removing some poisonous gases from the atmosphere. The more we express ourselves in our own environment, the more relaxed and happy we can be. Keeping the vibrations of your bedroom and everyday environment serene and confident will positively affect your mental well being, and in particular your sleeping pattern.

Noise Pollution

Noise is generally regarded as unwanted sound; it could be too loud, too persistent or just happen at the wrong time or without warning. People do adjust to the noise of living on main roads, near a railway or airport, and sometimes, even miss the noise when away from home. We have all heard someone say 'I can't sleep because it's too quiet'. It is common to encounter sleep disturbance when moving from one environment to another, be it from a quiet country village to a busy town near a main road or visa versa or when on holiday or away from home. It is best to keep the bedroom comfortable and quiet, but it maybe too quiet for you. Try running a fan or playing a radio softly in the background and see if that helps lull you to sleep. There are also devices available that generate 'white noise', sounds like the ocean surf or a steady rain, which can help 'quiet sensitive' people to sleep. (see useful addresses in appendix 1) Noise can be blocked out by double or triple glazing, but beware of an airless environment, a stuffy room can be as bad as a noisy one. If you are concerned about the noise coming from a neighbour's home, a local business or manufacturer, or noise from vehicles and equipment in the street, the best way to deal with the problem is to go to the source. If you cannot get satisfactory results from talking directly to those responsible, you can consider mediation. Go to your local authority and they will investigate the disturbance under the Environmental Protection Act 1990 (as amended by the Noise and Statutory Nuisance Act 1993).

Light pollution

The lights in your bedroom should be adjustable; bright when needed, sufficient for reading when required and low and subtle as desirable. Light pollution disturbances caused by external sources can be remedied by using thick lined curtains or efficient blinds, or both. Many people find that they sleep best in complete darkness, because of proximity to; car headlights, security lighting or bright street lighting, and may use a black out curtain, although this could bring problems waking up in the mornings if it is too dark. One solution to a very dark room is to buy and use a dawn simulator, which gradually increases the light intensity of some bedside lamps in a way that simulates natural dawn. (see appendix 1 for useful addresses) Avoid being disturbed by light while you sleep, this is especially important if you are a shift worker who is trying to sleep during the day.

BeÐroom Temperature

It is not possible to make rules for the correct temperature of the bedroom, as this will be different for every individual. There are many factors that will contribute to the sleeper being either too hot, or too cold; it will depend on what the sleeper is wearing, the type of bedclothes used, interior and exterior temperatures of the bedroom itself and devises used such hot water bottle and electric blanket. Another factor to be taken into account is one's sleeping partner; people generate heat and two people will generate more heat that one.

Cooler temperatures are generally more appropriate for bedrooms, but extremes should always be avoided. The bedroom should certainly be a few degrees cooler than other living areas and should be well aired, a temperature of between 16-18C (60-65F) suits many people, and makes a good starting point. If you air the bedroom thoroughly during the day, you will usually have enough fresh air for the night unless you have central healing turned full on in the bedroom, which is always a bad idea. Leave a window open during the day if possible and leave the bedroom door open for air to circulate through the house. Overheating impairs sleep because it takes the moisture out of the air, resulting in block airways, stuffiness and damage to the skin by drying it out. In summer try sleeping naked or in very light bedclothes between cotton sheets instead of in bedclothes and sheets and you will often be more comfortable. In winter, wear cozy bedclothes, switch on a safe electric blanket before bed, (do not leave an electric blanket on all night), or use a hot water bottle if needed. Bed socks will add that extra bit of warmth and comfort for those who get cold feet.

The Right Bed

If you do often find yourself tossing and turning, and unable to get comfortable, you may find that an uncomfortable or unsuitable bed is encumbering your night's sleep.

One of the first things you should think about when experiencing disturbed sleep, that appears to have no other logical reason, is your bed. A good new bed is a sound investment if it will help you sleep more easily and comfortably. Despite what is often said, a very firm mattress is not always appropriate. It is comfortable support that matters, and you should try out different mattresses before you buy a new bed. The right bed and pillows are very important for a good night's sleep, if you wake up with a stiff neck and aching back it would be a very good idea to check your bed comfort. So, how can you tell if your bed is past its best? Your mattress lifespan for offering the best support and comfort will vary depending on its quality, its frequency of use, the wear and tear it undergoes, and how well it has been looked after. A heavier person will need to change their mattress more frequently. As a rough guide, with normal use, you should change your mattress about every 10 years. Beds should be of medium firmness unless you have specific osteopathic problems, and your pillow must be firm enough to support your head and neck. Soft pillows do not support the neck allowing the head to flop to one side and the neck to be at an angle, which can cause tension in the neck and shoulders.

Consider hypoallergenic material, for pillows and mattresses, if you think dust mites could be a problem, as runny and stuffy noses or asthma, caused by dust mite allergy, are common causes of disturbed sleep. Many people find traditional Japanese futon beds very comfortable, they are filled with natural fabrics, layers of cotton wadding and the mattress lies on a slatted wooden base. The slatted base gives extra ventilation and the natural fibres are more friendly to asthma suffers and people with allergies. Futon mattresses need to be changed more frequently than conventional mattresses usually about every five years. (for information on bed comfort contact the sleep council addresses in appendix 1)

Beð Care

Proper care will keep your bed in good condition and contribute to restful sleep, always read and retain the manufacturer's care instructions and ask your retailer for advice. Air your bed and bed linen regularly, it is a good idea in the morning to pull back the covers and leave the mattress to breath for a few hours every day. The average person sweats half a pint of liquid each night and this goes into the mattress. Turn you mattress regularly, and vacuum your mattress and base from time to time to remove fluff, dust and mites. Don't make a habit of sitting on the side of the bed or letting the children use it as a trampoline. (see chapter 8 for more information on dust mites asthma and allergies)

Pets

I would recommend keeping animals of all kinds (cat and dog, or iguana) off the bed and out of the bedroom. This may be hard to do if you have already established a precedent, but with new pets train them to keep outside the bedroom door. Animals leave their fur, fleas, and skin flakes wherever they go, consider banning animals from the bedroom, particularly if you suffer from allergies or asthma. I know that many people are very comforted by having their faithful pet near them, on or in the bed; this must be something for the individual to decide.

Sleep Posture

The position adopted when preparing to sleep is very important. Sleeping with the head raised too high is often the cause of tension in the neck muscles, and of unsettled sleep.

Such a position, except when necessary for certain medical conditions, is also frequently the cause of headaches and actual disturbance in the skeletal structure of the upper spinal vertebrae. This can often arise when turning over in sleep while the head and neck are insufficiently supported and at unnatural angles. Some people can fall asleep in any position, but for most of us it is advisable to lie down on your side or back, with your spine aligned. If you sleep on your stomach it will be twisted, because your head will be on one side. Damage to posture caused during sleep can constitute cause for sleeplessness if neglected. Most stiffness arising from strain will pass off, but care should be taken to reduce or regulate the number of pillows and to get the right support for your neck.

Partners

In the west, the double bed is common, and couples usually sleep together, but if either party has a sleep problem that disrupts, or one of them snores or has restless leg syndrome. Two large single beds would probably be more sensible, you can always join your partner in his or her bed when you want some romance or a bit of company, and make it special. Sleeping together depends a great deal on the culture and affluence of the peoples concerned. In western society it is usual to have one's own bed and own bedroom to sleep in.

Creating A Bedtime Routine

An established routine is a good way to nurture satisfactory sleeping habits. Our biological clock is set to a sleep-awake routine and major changes in routine can have a negative effect. In this book I recommend a regular sleep routine and I have included a recommended checklist on page 115-118 for children and page 250 for genberal checklist. But this must never become overly obsessive and restricting or you will be making worse problems for yourself.

Chapter 3

Depression and Stress

Depression

Over two thirds of those who have trouble getting to sleep, or getting back to sleep, complain of an overactive brain, or of worry, stress and depression. We know that insomnia is often associated with depression, insomnia may be the first symptom of depression and it is likely that about half of all insomnia sufferers have some psychological cause to their sleep problems. If you have had major surgery, have had a key life shift such as divorce, bereavement, job change, recent move, or if you are just worried about something, you could experience some insomnia. The truth is that the fatigue you feel may not be sleep related, but stress related. If you feel despairing or suicidal, if you have lost interest or pleasure in things, if you have panic attacks, feelings of dread, palpitations or difficulty breathing you should go and see your doctor. If you are tense, suffer from headaches, stomach ache, anxiety or depression, then you probably need to work on stress reduction, for most people - sleep and mood are closely linked and can often lead to physical symptoms. If you suffer from a sleep disorder, this connection between how you feel and how well you sleep can be especially important and very significant to your overall health problems.

Depression is a disorder of mood, and can take the form of protracted and disproportionate melancholy and apathy. When someone experiences any type of sleep disturbance, it is important to see if there are any other symptoms of depression including depressed mood, loss of energy, irrational behaviour and suicidal tendencies. If disturbed sleep is a symptom of depression, then the situation may return to normal when the depression is satisfactorily treated.

Depressives tend to have trouble getting to sleep and wake in the early hours and find it impossible to get back to sleep. People with dementia are often afraid of the dark and this makes them confused and restless. Schizophrenics can be tortured by voices and pace up and down all night, while people with mania or compulsive behaviour are often hyper-active and don't sleep much at all. It would be possible to write a whole book just about stress and depression but that is not what I have set out to do I will however, in attempting to cover all aspects of insomnia suggest a few stress busting tactics and relaxation techniques in part three of this book.

Depression is not a weakness but an actual disorder that can be more disabling than many other ailments, because it makes the body susceptible to any weakness or disease that may come along. Sometimes it's difficult to separate actual clinical depression from sadness or melancholy. It is unfortunate that the term depression is used very casually, at times, to describe a feeling of mild irritation, or being a bit down. You can have the temporary blues when things don't go well for you if you lose your job, are ill, or at the end of a love affair. Most people will bounce back after a short while and feel no permanent depression.

Low dose anti-depressants are sometimes given for insomnia, but this is not recommended, if depression is truly present, then it will be inadequately treated, and if it is not present there are better alternative treatments for insomnia. Most commonly for depression doctors prescribe tranquilizers and anti-depressants, but these only numb the patient and do not help them face up to the underlying problems that are causing the depression in the first place. Psychotherapy can help to uncover the causes of depression and work out the problems that are involved.

Other therapies that can really help are Rosen method, aromatherapy and reflexology, there are also many natural herbal remedies you can take like St Johns Wort, (take care with St Johns Wort if you are taking any other medication, consult your doctor) it is also a very good idea to take some vitamin supplements, notably vitamin B complex, vitamin C and multimineral tablets. Many people suffering from depression also have low blood sugar or hypoglycemia it is a good idea to cut out sweet things and caffeine, they are a cause of the mood swings and sleeplessness that contribute to depression. (see part three for more details on complementary therapies) Women are more likely to develop depression than men this partly echoes women's fluctuating hormones, and depression is common during the menopause and after childbirth. However, these effects alone do not account for the imbalance between men and women.

There are some amino acids that can help some people suffering from depression; one of these is tyrosine, which helps activate the neurotransmitter norapinephrine, which helps to promote positive moods. People taking tyrosine have improved their sleeping patterns and psychological patterns in a very short space of time. Another amino acid is D-phenylalanine, which is also involved in epinephrine metabolism; D-phenylalanine is converted into tryrosine by the liver. One particular depression effects many people in the winter (SAD) seasonal affective disorder, and is caused by lack on sunlight.

Nutrition and Depression

There are many food related causes of depression, the most common being sub-optimum nutrition resulting in poor mental and physical energy. Disturbed blood sugar balance can result in periods of depression, people who produce excessive amounts of histamine are also prone to it. Adrenal exhaustion usually brought on by stress and over-use of stimulants can have this effect, food allergies too can bring on depression.

The brain produces a number of important chemicals (called neurotransmitters) that help control our mood and behaviour. They have names like serotonin, adrenaline, noradrenaline and dopamine. A deficiency of serotonin has been linked with depression. Drugs such as Prozac work by preventing the breakdown or removal of serotonin from the brain. The amino acid 5 hydroxy tryptophan helps prevent the breakdown of serotonin and can be taken as a supplement at night, it is very useful for children with headaches or sleep problems, and can be used to calm children with aggressive behaviour. St Johns Wort is a mild herbal anti-depressant that works in the same way as Prozac; it also inhibits the breakdown of serotonin. (see page 244 for more information about serotonin). However, there is evidence that depression may also result from the molecule dopamine. Dopamine gets turned into adrenaline, the substance that gets us going, and gives us our drive and enthusiasm. Taking the amino acid, tyrosine, will increase the dopamine metabolism. So tyrosine can also help relieve depression, and improve drive and enthusiasm. You should take tyrosine in the morning to get you up and moving, it also helps with obsessive and addictive tendencies, and will aid you in developing a healthy sleep pattern. (tyrosine is now only available by prescription)

Chronic Fatigue or ME

The condition post-viral syndrome, chronic fatigue syndrome or ME also know as 'myalgic encephalomyetlitis' and most insultingly 'yuppie flu'. It affects mostly teenagers, young adults and male and female professionals with hectic stressful lives. Once it was thought that it was a crippling, severe, persistent fatigue that lasted at least six months and dramatically reduced the ability to live a busy and active life. Now it is generally believed to follow viral infection, allergy, or dietary intolerance.

There are many causes of chronic fatigue, the most common of which is bad nutrition. The nutrients needed in energy production include vitamins C and B complex, iron and magnesium. Symptoms can include depression and extreme tiredness on exertion, and can result from the body's inability to detoxify being overloaded. It is advisable to see an ME specialist and nutrition consultant if you think you suffer from ME. Night sweats, and fevers are the most noticeable of the sleep disturbances which occur with this disease, waking up disorientated and with your head ringing from disturbing dreams can be another alarming symptom. Learning to enjoy these dreams, by relaxing into them can help you. (see relaxation techniques page 131)

Sleep in layers of bedclothes so you can throw back a top layer if you wake in a sweat. Then there are times when there is no good reason to wake up, you simply do. Whether or not you feel hungry or thirsty, you will often find that a very light snack or a hot drink will send you back to sleep quickly and safely. It will help regulate the blood sugar, hormone levels to the brain, calm the nervous and digestive systems. Always avoid sleeping-tablets unless there really is no other option. Disturbances of your sleep patterns are always unpleasant, many suffers of ME find that their illness throws their sleep patterns into total disarray, and they have continually to adjust their life styles to cope with irregular sleep needs. Sufferers usually find that they require more sleep than normal, but instead of taking it in one single block at night, their bodies tell them to rest at various points during the day. Make up your mind that while you are ill you will need to sleep at odd times of the day, but as you start to get better you can rest instead of sleep during the day, and this will gradually alter your sleep pattern to a more suitable rhythm.

Some chronic fatigue syndrome sufferers believe that trying to do too much too soon causes irreparable harm, so they lead a housebound or even bed-bound life. This reduces exercise tolerance and means that sufferers are even less able to live normally.

Many chronic fatigue syndrome sufferers find help in the complementary therapies, although no treatment, conventional or alternative works for everyone.

Overcoming chronic fatigue syndrome requires time and patience and there are no over night cures. (Contact the ME Association for further advice and information see useful addresses in appendix 1)

Mental Illness

In the UK one in four people seek help for mental problems at sometime during their lives, each year, 12 million people consult their doctor because they are depressed. Seven million people suffer from a serous mental disorder such as severe depression, phobia or schizophrenia. However, despite mental illness being more common than cancer, doctors often fail to recognize mental disorders and send people away with tranquillizers, antidepressants and sleeping pills. Not surprisingly, insomnia is caused by anxiety and depression and makes these diseases worse. In some cases, people suffering from depression may not realize that they are ill; depression can creep up on patients. Many other people regard depression as an appropriate reaction to life's events such as unemployment or bereavement; others may hope that the symptoms will just go away all by themselves. Major depression is serious; it undermines quality of life more than many other chronic diseases. Depression is a stifling feeling of not being able to cope, and in some cases, the intense mental torment drives patients to suicide, physical harm to others or self mutilation. Complementary therapies can really help the mentally ill by reinforcing their self-image and self worth and by balancing their internal energies.

Anxiety

Many people are prone to bouts of anxiety; they worry habitually, feel apprehensive, are constantly vigilant, many have difficulty concentrating and are easily startled. Exercise can help when feeling panicked, some brisk physical exercise will help release and regulate the hormones adrenaline and noradrenaline, which help maintain blood pressure. Avoid all caffeine where possible, excessive coffee and tea drinking can make matters worse by lowering blood sugar, and triggering the release of more adrenaline. Some people find that calcium supplements of one gram per day, plus magnesium up to 500 mg can reduce the frequency of panic attacks. Breath deeply and slowly, count to ten, some people prefer a re-breathing technique, with corrects the effects of hyperventilation. Place a paper bag over the nose and mouth, breath slowly in and out about ten times, remove the bag for a few minutes, and repeat if necessary. This has the effect of breathing back the carbon dioxide into the lungs, adjusting the acid in the blood, and calming down the nervous system.

The following extract is from the book *The Little Buddha*, from the story of the film by Bernardo Bertolucci staring Keanu Reeves as Prince Siddhartha.

In the story of the Buddha, when Prince Siddhartha had been meditating in silence in the wilderness for six years, he came one day to the river and lay down to sleep. Siddhartha had become so thin that by pressing his stomach he could feel his spine. He had not eaten anything but berries or the odd grain of rice for many years. It was early morning when he was awakened by the sound of a flute. An old man was teaching a young boy to play. He heard the old man tell the boy. "If you tighten the string too much, it will snap and if you leave it too slack, it won't play". This refers to the Buddhist philosophy of finding the middle way.

Phobias

A phobia is an abnormal or morbid fear or an aversion; phobias are fears out of all proportion to their cause. Some people are irrationally scared by spiders (arachnophobia), height, flying or open spaces (agoraphobia), and hypnophobia is the fear of sleeping.

Ironically, sufferers often recognize that their fears are unrealistic and irrational, but they feel they can do nothing about it. These fears and phobias can manifest themselves in the shape of dreams and nightmares. In the worst instances one may actually fear going to sleep there is a clinical condition where the patient fears that they may not wake up again if they go to sleep so they try to keep themselves awake. Most phobias that emerge in childhood disappear without treatment, but if they persist of first emerge in adult life they can be treated by counselling, natural remedies and hypnotherapy.

Obsessive-compulsive Disorder

Obsessions are persistent ideas, thoughts, impulses or routines that dominate some people's daily lives. An 'obsessive compulsive' person will have compulsions that are often repetitious actions performed to relieve the stress generated by an obsession. Examples can be: repeatedly checking that you have done something, washing hands over and over again, having to lay things out in exactly the same order or in the same position every time they do something. In this book I do recommend a regular bed time routine but going to bed at exactly the same time each day and with exactly the same

34

routine each time, like undressing in the same order i.e. right shoe, left shoe, and placing the shoes in exactly the same place each night, would be very unhealthy.

In the worst cases it can concern eating only the same type of food, or eating or drinking at the same time every day and can often ruin the persons relationships and rule their life. Anorexia and bulimia are conditions that could be called 'obsessive compulsive' disorders, in the worst of cases they can lead to death. (there will be more information about anorexia and bulimia in chapter 9)

Palpitations

Palpitations is an awareness of the heart beat, either because the heart is in fact beating more forcibly than usual or because the subject pays undue attention to it. Palpitation can happen at any time but many people can suffer from panic attacks and/or palpitations during the night. Nighttime palpitations can be very upsetting and badly disrupt sleep.

Chapter 4

Medication

There are numerous prescribed medications that can cause sleepless nights. Cold remedies that contain phenylporpanolamine (PPA), some blood pressure medications, appetite suppressants, Inderal and other beta blockers, and Dilantin for the prevention of seizures can all cause insomnia. Check with your doctor to see if any medications you are taking could interfere with your sleep, or check the label on the medicine itself.

Avoid taking nasal decongestants and other cold medications late in the day. While many ingredients in these preparations are known to cause drowsiness, they can have the opposite effect on some people and act as a stimulant. Always discuss your sleep problems with your doctor along with other medical problems and talk over the best time to take any regularly prescribed medications. You should always inform your doctor if you are taking any herbal remedies or alternative medicines of any kind and plan to use other complementary therapies, so that they do not interfere with your treatment.

Prescribed Medication

In the long run, sleeping pills, especially barbiturates, are apt to make insomnia worse rather than better. There are no prescribed sleeping pills that foster ordinary sleep patterns naturally. They work by knocking out the awake centers of the brain, which causes sleep, but of an unsatisfactory quality. Sleeping pills should never be used continually, or over long periods of time. Some pills abolish the deepest stage of Non Rapid Eye Movement (NREM) sleep. And most suppress much needed rapid Eye Movement (REM) sleep, which is the kind during which most dreams occur, and we need to dream. Sleeping pills, such as barbiturates, have been found to be less effective than tranquillizers. Minor tranquillizers may be used for a few nights to restore the sleep cycle and to reduce anxiety, but they are not meant as a long-term treatment.

The pharmacological effect of barbiturates wears off after two weeks because the body learns to tolerate them. Sleeping pills can also become addictive and as the effects wear off it becomes necessary to take more pills to get the same result. Currently the most effective therapy is to identify any problems that may be preventing sleep and to attempt to solve them, meanwhile reducing the person's anxiety about the insomnia itself.

Large numbers of people take, or attempt to take, their lives by the use of sleeping drugs. Research has shown the responsibility for the increase in attempted suicides on the freer prescribing of sleeping drugs under the National Health Service. I do believe that some of the cases of attempted suicide by barbiturate drugs are unintentional. The victim takes one or two tablets to obtain sleep and then, while only partly awake, and with most senses dulled by the medications already taken, swallows a second and fatal dose. The combination of alcohol and sleeping pills or other medications can also be a lethal recipe for the vulnerable. Under present-day circumstances, and despite the warnings of doctors and chemist, it is easy for people to accumulate absolutely lethal stocks of drugs. In fact, it is too easy, and one wonders that there are not more incidents. Practically all sleeping drugs have deadly properties, they are very dangerous to have around, and it is much too easy to take an overdose. It must be reiterated, too, that drugs never get at the cause of insomnia; they merely provide a night's sleep often at the cost of digestive disorders, headaches and acid bloodstream, and the possibility of sustaining an addiction to drugs.

Drugs can never generate true relaxation and relaxation is essential to natural sleep.

Sleeping Pills

Sleeping pills can help provide sounder sleep and can improve alertness the following day but this relief is only temporary, since sleeping pills are not a cure for insomnia. For some types of insomnia, breathing disorders for example, sleeping pills can be very dangerous. Always avoid taking prescribed sleeping pills or any over the counter sleep aids with alcohol. Barbiturates should only be used for severe intractable insomnia. They produce tolerance, liability to abuse and severe withdrawal effects similar to those seen with alcohol abstinence. Their margin of safety is very narrow and severe toxic effects leading to coma and death are common following overdose or enhancement by alcohol they induce hepatic microsomal enzymes thereby affecting the rate of elimination and hence the effects on many drugs that are metabolised by the liver.

Benzodiazephines act by protentiating the action of the widespread inhibitory neurotransmitter, GABA, thereby dampening neuronal activity in the brain. They are widely used as hypnotics because of their lower incidence of adverse effects and their safety in overdose relative to the barbiturates. However, the longer acting compounds can induce residual sedative effects the next day, and can accumulate especially in the elderly. Discontinuation, particularly of the shorter acting compounds, may be attended by rebound insomnia after short-term use and withdrawal phenomena after longer-term use. Because of this risk of dependence, they should only be used to treat insomnia, which is severe, disabling or causing intolerable distress. Even so, treatment should be short term, i.e. less that 2 weeks, and preferably intermittent.

(extract from MIMS monthly index of medical specialties)

Benzodiazephines, the most notorious being Valium and Ativan, were introduced in the 1960's as a supposedly safer alternative to the acknowledged habit forming barbiturates and since then have become the most widely prescribed drugs in the world.

Short-acting sleeping pills are designed to last long enough to benefit sleep but leave the body quickly to minimise sleepiness the next day. Short acting drugs include temazepam (restoril), triazolam (Halcion), and zolpidem tartrate (Ambien). The long-acting flurazepam (Dalmane) is more likely to make you drowsy the following day, and is more often used for illness or anxiety states that require daytime sedation. Triazolam (Halcion), one of the most popular prescription sleeping medications in the US, can cause mental confusion and even amnesia. There have also been reports that the use of drugs such as temazepam (Restoril), secobarbital (Seconal), flurazepam (Dalmane), and diazepam (Valium) may lead to confusion, sluggishness, restlessness, and heightened anxiety, as well as prolonged sedation and drug dependency. People who take sleeping pills are more likely to have accidents from drowsiness in automobile accidents and industrial mishaps.

Withdrawal from Prescribed Medications

Withdrawal from prescribed medication, in particular anti-depressants, sleeping pills and traquillisers can sometimes be very tough, and will often cause insomnia itself for a time while the body adjusts to its natural rhythm. When proposing to come off sleeping pills, plan for the correct time, don't try to do it when you are stressed, moving house or changing your job. Make sure you tell family and friends what you are doing and ask for their help and support.

Breaking the Sleeping Pill Habit

Tests have shown that sleeping pills disrupt normal sleeping patterns. All sleeping drugs suppress paradoxical (rapid eye movement, REM) sleep but when these drugs are stopped paradoxical sleep increases. As paradoxical sleep is associated with dreaming, withdrawal of sleeping drugs may result in restless sleep with dreaming and nightmares. These withdrawal effects make the individual think that he/she is unable to sleep without sleeping drugs, not realizing that the drug's effects have produced the disturbed sleep.

If you have been taking sleeping drugs nightly for weeks, months or years and wish to stop them you must reduce the dose very slowly over several weeks. Therefore it is better to consult your doctor who will give you a small-dose preparation to help you do this. A gradual reduction in dosage over several weeks may enable you to break a sleeping-drug habit. But you will have some restless nights until your brain gets used to sleep without drugs. One factor that causes insomnia in withdrawal is high adrenaline levels, which cause dreams and nightmares. There may also be muscle and joint problems, itching and burning skin and bowel problems. Please try some of the remedies for insomnia that I have outlined in this book until your find what is right for you. But if you are trying to withdraw from any prescribed drug always do it with the help and support of a qualified health practitioner, and inform them of any therapies or natural remedies you intend to use. (see useful addresses in appendix 1 for help with coming off tranquillizers, sleeping pills and anti-depressants.)

Chapter 5

Sleep Disorders

What are sleep disorders? Some can occur while asleep without waking up the sufferer, others cause you to wake up and suffer from broken sleep or insomnia. According to the American Sleep Disorders Association there are some 84 disorders of sleeping and waking that result in diminished quality of life and personal health, and jeopardize public safety because of their role in traffic and industrial accidents. These include problems with staying awake or staying with a regular sleep-awake cycle, sleepwalking, bed-wetting, nightmares, restless legs syndrome, snoring and sleep apnoea syndrome.

Some sleep disorders are potentially fatal. Sleepiness causes accidents, possible 30 to 50 per cent of all traffic accidents are the result of sleepiness, and sleepiness is very often a specific factor in fatal accidents. (according to a RAC report) Sleepiness reduces productivity, impedes social skills, creates negative feelings, dulls the healing process, obstructs the immune system and promotes lethargy and depression. About one in seven people have insomnia that is severe enough to affect their lives or health, and one in eleven have insomnia almost every night for over six months at a time.

Sleep problems affect health and well-being in one of two ways: sleep problems cause sleepiness, either directly or as a direct result of disrupted sleep, and this sleepiness can then lead to accidents and poor performance; second, disrupted sleep can damage some basic life functions, such as circulation and digestion.

What Is Snoring

Snoring is defined as a coarse sound made by vibrations of the soft palate and other tissue in the mouth, nose and throat (upper airway). It is caused by a partial blockage of the upper airway and the nature of that blockage must be identified before the snoring can be treated or cured. When asleep we lose all muscle tone, which creates a narrowing of the airway. During waking hours muscle tone keeps the airway in good shape, that's why we don't snore when we are awake. The reduction of breathing space during sleep is the pre-condition for snoring. But snorers have an additional feature; an obstruction of some kind, somewhere between the adams-apple and the tip of the nose. This blockage can be from swollen tissue, congestion or a deformity. Very overweight people may be prone to snoring because when they relax in

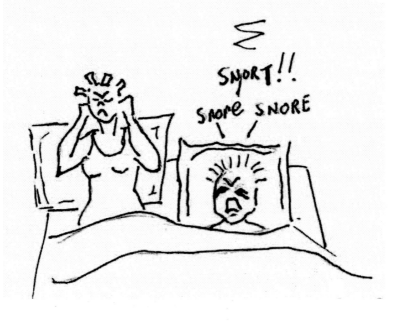

sleep their extra weight presses down on the larynx and throat and impedes normal breathing. Snoring can often be the result from overindulgence in some of life's pleasures like food and alcohol. The following are causes, and by moderating them, the snorer can often become quieter and more comfortable at night:

• Smoking
Smoking irritates the lining of the nasal cavity and throat causing swelling and catarrh. The likelihood of snoring is increased as more cigarettes are smoked, the nasal passage becomes congested nasal breathing is impaired and airflow through the nose is decreased. Even passive smoking can cause chronic inflammation of the nose and throat passages, thus increasing the risk of snoring.

• Over Eating
Over eating and/or lack of exercise can lead to an increase in fat around the throat. You may also lose the muscle tone needed to keep the airway open sufficiently at night to allow normal breathing, and the narrow airway is more likely to vibrate. Weight loss with accompanying fat reduction will certainly help to alleviate snoring, and may help with stress related problems, as you will also have more energy and your general health may well improve.

• Alcohol
Alcohol can exacerbate snoring, alcohol travels to all areas of the body and slows the brain's responses, causing the muscles to relax. Alcohol also acts as a depressant and increases feeling of stress and tension. The relaxation of the muscula-ture causes the top of the throat or pharynx to collapse inducing snoring.

Alcohol can induce obstructive sleep apnoea in those who are otherwise just snorers. As with smoking, alcohol causes nasal airway irritation, which increases the airway resistance when breathing. The consumption of alcohol affects every organ and system in the body, it can damage heart tissue and elevate blood pressure. It also has a high caloric content, and people who are heavy drinkers are often overweight.

• Sleeping pills
Sleeping tablets increase the state of relaxation by knocking you out straight into deep sleep, which can also lead to snoring

• Sleeping position
Sleeping position is very important for snorers, while sleeping on you back your tongue, your chin and any excess fatty tissue under your chin will probably relax back and squash your airway causing snoring. It would be better for people who snore to sleep on their side.

• Dust and house dust mites
Dust mite droppings can cause allergies and nasal congestion similar to the symptoms displayed by those individuals who smoke. They will cause stuffed noses that will add to difficulty in breathing and exacerbate snoring.

Singing or exercising your voice for 20 minutes a day could cure your snores, according to studies at the University of Exeter. Singing helps tone up the throat muscles, making them less likely to vibrate during sleep.

Sleep Apnoea
Sleep apnoea is a condition, which stops you breathing when you are asleep; the cessation of breathing automatically forces you to wake up in order to start breathing again. This can happen many times during the night, making it hard for your body to get enough oxygen, and preventing you from obtaining enough good quality sleep. There are three types of sleep apnoea, which are caused by different factors:

1. Obstructive Sleep Apnoea (OSA) is the most common form. It is the result of structures in the throat blocking the flow of air in and out of the lungs during sleep.

2. Central Sleep Apnoea (CSA) is a condition when the brain does not send the right signals to tell you to breathe when you are asleep. In other words the brain 'forgets' to make you breathe.

3. Mixed sleep Apnoea is a combination of both OSA and CSA.

People who have sleep apnoea may experience some of the following symptoms:

Loud heavy snoring, often interrupted by pauses and gasps, waking up at night suddenly gasping for breath, which lead to; daytime sleepiness, decreased daytime alertness, loss of energy, irritability, short temper, morning headaches, forgetfulness, changes in mood or behaviour, anxiety or depression, decreased interest in sex. There are obvious risks for asthmatics and people with other respiratory problems. High blood pressure, heart disease, and increased risk of stroke are all associated with sleep apnoea.

Sleep Hypopnoea

Sleep Hypopnoea is a decrease of airflow during sleep because of a partial blocking of the airway (obstructive hypopnoea/ snoring) or less effort being put forward to breath (central hypopnoea). (For help with snoring and sleep apnoea problems see useful addresses in the appendix 1)

Night Terrors

A night terror is a single or reoccurring, frightening image seen in deep sleep, abruptly awakening a person bolt upright sometimes with a piercing scream followed by behaviour of intense fear which, can include thrashing, kicking, shaking. They are usually brought on by 'post traumatic stress syndrome' or after a traumatic experience, often reported in children for no apparent reason; they are sometimes caused by unexplained events of fears of which we are not always aware.

RLS (Restless Leg Syndrome) Ekbom Syndrome

RLS is a disagreeable or annoying sensation in the legs usually occurring during the day or before sleep begins. It causes an almost irresistible urge to move the legs leading to restlessness and discomfort that can wake you up and stop you falling asleep. RLS is mainly associated with elderly women but it can also affect men and children and there is evidence to suggest that it runs in families. The first symptoms may occur mildly or infrequently in the teenage years, occur again in pregnancy to fade way after birth only to reappear later in life. Studies have shown an association with stress, depression and anxiety. It is known that about a third of all patients with rheumatoid arthritis also suffer from this condition.

PLMD (Periodic Limb Movement Disorder)

PLMD is involuntary leg, arm or body twitches during sleep sometimes brought on by disagreeable or annoying sensations, which feels like a crawling feeling on the surface of the skin, for no apparent reason. People may not awaken fully and may not even be aware of them except that they will be restless and move about more in their sleep. (In chapter 7

there is more about RLS and PLMD in relation to prolonged
bed rest and illness).

Idiopathic Insomnia

Idiopathic describes any disease or condition of unknown
cause or that spontaneously and repeatedly occurs. Idiopathic
insomnia is also known as childhood onset insomnia, it is a
lifelong inability to get adequate sleep and reflects an under-
active sleep system or an over-active awake system. The
mental state of the sufferer usually remains fairly good. There
are no apparent events that are a stimulus and the person
remains alert and coherent most of the time unless other
factors come into play.

Narcolepsy

Narcolepsy is an inherited disease causing fits of sleepiness
and drowsiness. It usually develops in late adolescence or
early adulthood, and is caused by an over-active sleep system,
over which the person has no control. It is a rare disorder and
the patient is normal except for fits of uncontrollable
sleepiness and sudden waves of muscular weakness.
Hallucinations can occur at sleep onset, this is caused by the
confusion of not knowing if you are awake or dreaming.
Amphetamines and similar drugs are generally used to ward
off attacks. Taking naps during the day reduces the need to
sleep and so lessens the number of episodes of uncontrolled
sleep. Attacks are often triggered by strong emotions, such as
joy or anger. Some narcoleptics have a problem sleeping at
night and keep waking flushed, agitated and with a rapid
heart beat. It can be very dangerous if someone has an attack
in the wrong circumstances i.e. while driving or during some
other some kind of activity where they might hurt themselves
or others.

Cataplexy

Cataplexy is the sudden weakening experienced by narcoleptics when emotional: (knees buckling, speech slurring, head bowing, collapsing but remaining awake) lasting from a few seconds to several minutes.

Needing to go to the Bathroom in the Night, Nocturia

In most healthy sleep, and under usual circumstances, urination at night occurs once or not at all. There can be many reasons for needing to go to visit the toilet more than usual. Frequent nocturia disrupts sleep and may indicate other problems that are damaging the quality of your sleep. A weak bladder due to a urinary complaint or a condition such as cystitis can cause frequent urinating and some discomfort, (see page 131 on cystitis) but an access of alcohol can also cause problems. Limit the amount you drink within an hour or two of bedtime and always go to the toilet just before you go to bed whether you need to or not. If you have obstructive sleep apnoea it is often linked with other symptoms including nocturia. Avoid diuretic foods such as watermelon, and caffeinated drinks such and tea, coffee and colas in the late evening. If you are taking water pills (diuretic medications) ask you doctor if they can be taken early in the day and not late afternoon and evening.

Sleeping Sickness

Sleeping sickness, trypanosomiasis, is an infectious disease confined to tropical Africa, transmitted by tsetse flies. West African sleeping sickness is due to Trypanosama Gambiense, and is transmitted by the bite of a tsetse fly, Glossina palpalis, these fly breeds in damp forest near riverbanks, and bites man for choice. Often the patient sleeps little, but day and night he is dull and apathetic. The patient may starve for want of the energy to eat, or die of any passing infection. This disease is confined to the belt of rain forest along the West African coast and through the Congo basin to the Great Lakes. The basic problem of treatment is that the patient often never gets the drugs that will help him, but if he does, it can be helped if caught in the early stages.

Chagas' Disease

Chagas' disease the South American trypanosomiasis is due to T. cruzi, and is transmitted in the excreta of various bugs. After the initial fever, Chagas' disease often runs a fairly harmless course, unless it invades muscle and other tissue. If this happens to the heart, the disease if fatal and there are no effective drugs to treat Chagas' disease.

Sleepy Sickness

Encephalitis lethargica is an epidemic virus infection, it was a widespread epidemic in the closing years of the First World War and after some time just came to an end. It was also known as 'sleepy sickness' but is nothing to do with African sleeping sickness. Many of its victims were left with a severe disturbance of muscular co-ordination (post-encephaltic parkinsomism). At the time there was no known way to isolate the virus, and after about 1923 the disease vanished. But everything about the epidemic suggests a virus infection. Historically, it is an interesting example of a serious disease that has appeared from nowhere and mysteriously departed, like some of the plagues of antiquity.

Sleepwalking or Somnambulism

Somnambulism stems from Somnus, the Roman god of sleep, and is one of many English words derived from classical mythology. Somnambulism combines somnu, 'sleep', and Ambulare, 'to walk'. Related words are somniloquy, which means talking in one's sleep and blends somnus with loqui, somniferous, 'inducing sleep', somnolent, 'feeling sleepy', and insomnia, 'without sleep'. People can sleep walk for many reasons, they could be restless because they are sleeping on a ley line, (see page 137) or they may have a worry or trauma that is upsetting their sleep. Sleepwalking is usually harmless if the person does not wander out into the street or in front of traffic. A sleepwalker should not be woken up while sleepwalking, but should be gently guided back to bed and kept out of harmful situations.

Sleep Talking, Somniloquy

Sleep talking is not usually harmful, unless the sleeper gets verbally abusive or the speech is combined with actions that could harm himself/herself or others. It may indicate unusually deep or unusually disrupted sleep.

Violence or other Activity in sleep

Violent movements can occur as a result of exaggerated comfort movements, stretching, sexual arousal, thrashing around during sleep terrors, sleep walking and different kinds of nocturnal epilepsy, sleep apnoea episodes or dreaming and acting out dreams. Screaming, shouting or groaning in your sleep is a harmless, if often annoying phenomenon, particularly to sleeping partners. Don't ever underestimate the danger of violence during sleep, many people have been harmed or even murdered by their partners while enacting violent dreams. If you, or someone you are close to has the potential for violence in their sleep, be it from sleepwalking or dream enacting, this person should sleep alone in a separate room until the problem is resolved. Acting out our dreams can be harmless, unless the dreamer is under threat himself or herself or threatening someone in their dream, where this violence could spill out and onto the person's sleeping partner. Sexual arousal is a frequent occurrence in dreams and not harmful in itself, unless the sleeper becomes over active, amorous or demonstrative to their unwilling sleeping partner. Seek help from your doctor or a sleep specialist if you or someone you care for is in danger of hurting themselves or others in their sleep movement, dream enactment, or if sleep walking or sleep talking is seriously disturbing sleep. If any of these conditions have come on suddenly, become more frequent or developed into a serious difficulty it would be advisable to get some expert advise on how to deal with the underlying problems that are causing the disturbances.

Night Eating Syndrome

Night Eating Syndrome is a condition brought on by stress. The person gets up in the night to eat, usually high carbohydrate snacks, sometimes two of three times each night. It can be helpful to leave a drink and a dry biscuit or some grapes by the side of the bed, so that the person can have a bite to eat without disturbing their sleep too much.

Psycho-physiological Insomnia

Psycho-physiological insomnia is also known as learned or conditioned insomnia. As with other chronic insomnia it is brought on in susceptible individuals after some traumatic event or stressful period in their life. There is usually one point that triggers the insomnia, but there are usually other factors associated with chronic insomnia, which, sustain the condition. These may originate as result of trying to cope with the sleeplessness and deal with an on going problem at the same time. Napping is not necessarily the wrong thing to do in this situation, though chronic insomniacs often cannot take naps, whatever keeps them awake at night can also keep them awake at day. Conditioned insomniacs will react to stress by getting increased muscle tension, which makes it difficult to fall asleep. (Exercise can often help see chapter 15)

TMJ, Sleep Bruxism or Tooth-grinding

Bruxism is the involuntary or habitual grinding or clenching of the teeth that will often disturb sleep and cause headaches. Bruxism may start in babies and children when teeth first grow, and continue into adolescence. It is also very common with the elderly who have false teeth that are loose fitting or not fitted properly, if they are not taken out at night. People suffering stress and nervous tension will often grind their teeth, teeth grinding is also one of the most common causes of headaches. When bruxism occurs in sleep it is often accompanied by slow eye movements and sometimes twitching and will certainly lead to restless sleep. There are night-guards that can be worn to protect the teeth, also see your dentist to check that there are no alignment problems. A good therapy for relieving tooth grinding is Indian Head Massage, (see pages 176-177) and try to sleep on your back so that your jaw is more relaxed than it is lying on your side or stomach where your face is under pressure.

Advanced Sleep Phase Syndrome, (ASPS)

The tendency to be 'early to bed early to rise', which is inclined to develop with more elderly people. ASPS can disrupt a person's social life, since it is frustrating to be awake early in the morning while others are still sleeping, and difficult to stay awake later in the evening when others are engaged in social activities. People with ASPS often try various strategies to stay up later. Even if they are successful in pushing back bedtime, however, they may not be able to sleep any later since their body clocks still awaken them early. Treatments for ASPS include light timing lamps that can stimulate the sleep/wake cycle and cause a delay in the feeling of sleepiness in the early evening, and can also postpone early morning awakening.

Napping

A nap is any short sleep episode that occurs outside the main sleep period, it can supply primary sleep. Naps can be planned, going to bed for an hour after lunch or when sick, or unplanned, dozing in front of the television at night. Naps can be refreshing and restore alertness, but a nap in mid-afternoon will probably make it harder for you to sleep at night. Elderly people often have a problem with this, and daytime naps should be avoided where possible. Very long naps have all the characteristics of shortened regular sleep and should, on the whole, be avoided by people with a regular sleep schedule unless the person is ill or recovering from a lack of normal sleep. No matter how tired you may feel during the day, unless you're very sick or have experienced some major disruption of your schedule, don't nap. If you feel sleepy during the daytime, try to get some fresh air go for a walk outside, if possible, have a cold drink, or do something specific to keep your mind alert. People who are ill, disabled or bedridden will often have problems with sleeping during the day and then not being able to sleep at night, particularly if they are in pain or have to take regular medication. It can help to try to keep the mind active during the day, read if possible, do a crossword, listen to the radio, television, music, or story tapes to keep the mind active and awake during the daytime even if you are not able to undertake more active activities.

Many cultures do have a short sleep, or siesta during the afternoon, this is often to escape the hottest part of the day, and then they will go to bed much later in the evening. We have a low energy period between 3-5 in the afternoon when the body often needs a rest, this can be a low blood sugar period that can be remedied by having something light to eat with a drink, glass of fruit juice, banana, handful of nuts, or a biscuit with a cup of tea. Naps if required, when you are ill, or adjusting to new time zone, should be intended as light refreshment, and not a substitute for nighttime sleep. They should not last longer than 30 minutes, otherwise you go into deep sleep, from which it may be hard to wake up and you are likely to feel worse than when you went to sleep, i.e. drowsy, dry mouthed and heavy limbed.

Jet Lag

Jet lag is a good example of how things can go wrong with the biological clock, moving to a new time zone faster than the body can adapt. It will cause problems in getting to sleep and staying awake out of the normal sleep wake cycle.Long plane trips leave you feeling dry mouthed, gritty and irritable. Many individuals find it difficult to sleep on planes and it is often the recourse to eat and drink too much, while at the same time staying inactive. the best thing to do is eat little, drink plenty of water, avoid alcohol, keep your skin moist, and try to stretch your legs every hour. Rosemary oil on a handkerchief inhaled on the flight or in the bath will help after flying. Then try to adjust to the new time zone as swiftly as possible by re-

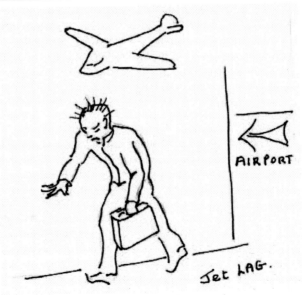

AIRPORT

Jet LAG.

setting your watch when you start your journey. Exercise can help some people before and after the flight, you should certainly get up a few times and have a good stretch during the flight. If it is possible fly by day rather than night, and try to adjust to the new time zone as quickly as possible when you arrive by eating and sleeping straight away in the correct time for the new time zone. Don't go to bed as soon as you get to your destination, if you can go out and get some fresh air, preferably in the sun. Have a high carbohydrate meal with plenty of fruit and vegetables, and avoid heavy proteins until the following day. The hormone melatonin is helpful to fight jet lag. Take one capsule for three nights before the flight, the day you travel and three days afterwards, before you go to bed.

Shift Work

Shift work can be a problem for many people, adapting to night work or shift work at different times of day can play havoc with your sleep. If you are a night worker who wants to sleep well in the morning, avoid bright light on the way home from work. Wear dark glasses, providing they don't make you too sleepy or obscure your view.

Vocational professions such as nursing, the police and the fire service all require adjustments to sleeping routines to those who work in them. Other people, such flight staff on an aeroplane, can find their lives very disrupted when sleep patterns are constrained or disturbed without regular routine. Light and noise is often a real problem, bedrooms are often not adequately shielded. Double or triple glazing, double blinds and thicker doors can all improve sleep perseverance and quality. One of the most important things is to stand by you habitual pre-sleep routine. If you are hungry at the end of a shift before going to bed eat lightly and drink a glass of water or herb tea, no caffeine, have a larger meal when you get up. Some people find it beneficial to take a short nap, exercise or have a high carbohydrate meal before their shift starts. Try to work in bright, preferably full-spectrum light and don't drink alcohol, especially before going to work.

The homeopathic remedy Cocculus 30c can be good for insomnia from a disturbed sleep pattern or shift work.

Chapter 6

Recreational Drugs and Stimulants

Not Poppy, nor mandragora,
Nor all the drowsy syrups of the world,
Shall ever medicine thee to that sweet sleep
Which thous owedst yesterday
Othello, William Shakespeare.

Caffeine stimulates the nervous system and adrenaline production, this will keep you awake and hyperactive. The disadvantageous effects of caffeine can last for up to 14 hours. Recreational drugs, such as cannabis, disrupt sleep patterns by depressing the central nervous system, while amphetamines have a stimulating effect, Many prescription drugs e.g. anti histamines and diuretics can also disturb sleep, talk to your GP about alternatives and correct times to take medications. For example diuretics can be taken in the morning rather than the evening.

Alcohol

Alcohol when used in moderation and used socially can sometimes reduce anxiety and help promote sleep, but it does not cause sleep it reduces sleepiness. The rate of alcoholism in insomniacs is twice that of good sleepers, and many alcoholics endeavour to use alcohol as a sleep aid, with the result that an estimated 10 per cent of alcoholism is a consequence of insomnia.

Alcohol impairs breathing and therefore often causes further breathing problems for people afflicted with sleep apnoea. Men of middle years who snore and who get sleepy during the day should not use alcohol to try and sleep. Headaches in the morning are often not only the result of alcohol but of impaired breathing and de-hydration. Alcohol is a diuretic, this means you urinate more and can be disturbed in the night when you have to get up to go to the toilet. Alcohol promotes sleepiness and so even a little alcohol can be treacherous for a sleepy person who is driving late at night. However, don't use alcohol to help you to get to sleep, because it seriously damages the quality of sleep. It may even cause you to wake up or stir after an hour or two with signs of arousal such as sweating, headache, dry mouth, a racing heart and/or restlessness. In general, it is considered healthier to restrict alcohol consumption to no more than 4 units, (two pints of beer), a day for male, and 2 units a day for females. Alcohol contains a lot of calories, and while reasonable consumption (one glass of red wine per day) appears to give some protection for some heart and circulatory problems, more than the equivalent to three or four alcoholic drinks a day would seem to increase blood pressure for many.

Nicotine

Nicotine both stimulates and relaxes, but is not consistently useful in aiding alertness. Nicotine stimulates the nervous system and triggers adrenaline release. Some research shows that smokers tend to have lighter, more broken sleep than non smokers and that they feel heavier and more sluggish first thing in the morning. If you do smoke, never smoke in bed, or if you wake up during the night. Apart from anything else, the risk of dropping a lighted cigarette and setting fire to the bed or house is great.

Nicotine in cigarettes, cigars and tobacco is addictive and causes respiratory problems as well as many other health problems like cancer, poor nutrition and impaired immunity. In addition to causing dry and discoloured skin, unhealthy smell to cling to your clothes and skin and bad breath. Withdrawal can be difficult, but giving up is worth the effort if it will help improve the quality of your sleep, get help if needed. Weight gain is not inevitable if you replace smoking with other more healthy activities. Withdrawal is associated with headaches and sleeplessness but usually these effects will soon pass. Try to increase the time between cigarettes, preferably by at least half as much again, have no smoking zones in the house, and never smoke in the bedroom and preferably not the car. Seek out alternatives to the places or situations that encourage you to smoke the most, and think about what you can do with all that extra money in your pocket each week, maybe that special holiday you have always wanted or a better standard of living for you and your loved ones. Enroll the help of friends and loved ones and think of your health and of those around you, you will have more energy, be healthier and more able to fight off disease. Passive smoking does almost as much harm as active smoking, always be aware of the feelings and senses of non-smokers. Never smoke around children, not only does it damage their health, stunt their growth, it creates a very bad role model and example for their own behaviour.

Marihuana, Hemp, Cannabis or Grass

Marihuana, marijuana or cannabis may relax you when you first use it, but eventually it will make sleep more difficult and can make you over anxious. The active compounds of marihuana are an alkaloid; tetrahydrocannabinol (THC) and its effects are a sense of well being, escape from reality, and hallucinations. But as with alcohol and other drugs affecting mood, the effect is much influenced by the circumstances in which it is taken. It may aid anxiety in the short term by relaxing the nervous system, and thus cause sleepiness but the results lessen with long-term use. About a third of regular users suffer from mild anxiety, depression, or irritability, all of which interfere with sleep. Some users have severe anxiety, panic attacks, and paranoia, delusions or hallucinations and a number of regular marihuana users have sustained brain damage.

Amphetamines (speed)

Amphetamine is a drug related to adrenaline, it is used to combat lethargy and depression, it stimulates the adrenal system and it will keep you awake.

Amphetamine, which has taken the place of cocaine among drugs of addiction, can injure the heart and cause serious mental derangement if taken habitually.

Amphetamine withdrawal is associated with increased sleepiness as well as increased REM during sleep, and it can cause nightmares.

Cocaine and Crack

Cocaine is an alkaloid stimulant that produces euphoria its effects are similar to adrenaline, stimulating the heart. It is a notorious drug of addiction, causing temporary elation and hallucinations, habitual use causes grave deterioration of personality and sometimes insanity. It works through the brain messenger dopamine, which is involved in the control of movement and wakefulness. Cocaine withdrawal is associated with sleepiness. Crack is a concentrated, highly addictive form of cocaine.

Heroin

Diamorphine, Diacetyl morphine is a synthetic derivative or morphine intended to have pain killing properties, it turned out to be very addictive. Heroin affects the pattern of sleep stages, but is most disturbing when it is discontinued. Intense nightmares may occur on withdrawal, this is called cold turkey.

Ecstasy

Ecstasy makes you very relaxed and loving, often more sexually aware and intimate with those around you. It is often used at raves and parties where the goal is to stay up all night, it also dehydrates the body and you have to drink more fluids and it will keep you awake.

Solvent Abuse

Many common solvents, such as those used in glue for model aeroplanes, are chemically related to anaesthetics such as ether and chloroform, or to alcohol. Like these they are intoxicating. Inhaling the vapour of certain glue solvents causes fleeting excitement followed by confusion, dizziness and stupor. If, as easily happens, 'glue sniffing' becomes a habit, the brain is liable to be permanently damaged along with the kidneys, liver, lungs and heart.

Drugs and alcohol can also trigger nightmares; nightmares often follow a bad trip or an excess of alcohol. Bad dreams or nightmares can force us to confront issues with which we have refused to deal, and they can sometimes contain a message that demands to be heard. If the subconscious mind is influencing our dreams to such an extent, it is trying desperately to attract our attention to a particular issue. It may well be healthier to deal with the issue raised than recoiling away from them by using the crutch of drugs and stimulants.

Chapter 7

Illnesses and Bed Confinement

Many routine medical problems affect healthy sleep, whether through disturbance as a result of pain or discomfort, or more directly. Research has shown that people naturally enjoy more deep, low wave sleep when recovering from illness or an operation, and that this kind of sleep speeds up the healing process. Sometimes sleep problems can be a sign of a physical problem like an over active thyroid, which produces too much of the hormone thryoxine. (see page 96) This increases your metabolic rate so that your system goes into overdrive and your heart races, which makes it hard to sleep. Research shows that sleeping more during times of infectious illness help us fight the infection and recover more quickly. Many people have gone to bed feeling ill and feverish and woken refreshed and well, sleeping seems to help in fighting disease.

Over-sleepiness is a natural consequence of practically all infectious diseases. This may be due to the effect of the body's immune system increasing production of certain protein and antibodies in response to the infection. Sleep may play a role in helping us to resist infection; lack of sleep depletes levels of white blood cells essential for fighting infections, and one of the body's main defence systems. Ill health, whether it is caused by chronic or serious conditions, injury, or by any other common complaint, is one of the main causes of disrupted sleep.

Pain, particularly, makes it difficult to get to sleep, and it can reduce the amount of deep sleep because it unsettles, resulting in broken sleep and restlessness because of difficulty in getting comfortable. Sleep disorders can kill, studies have shown that up to three times the rate of strokes and five times the rate of heart attacks occur in people with poor sleep. This is not just among the old or disabled, younger people are similarly afflicted.

Why does sleep, or the lack of sleep, affect the heart and circulation? Many people with poor sleep have breathing problems such as snoring or sleep apnoea. Also sleep disruption is stressful, and stress reactions take their toll on any other factors like heart disease and any chronic disease or ailment. Sleep is the restorer, our bodies are renewing themselves while we rest, when our sleep is disrupted we lose our restful, restorative hours of sleep, this is almost like growing older faster. There are other health issues, which might not be as lethal as the heart and circulation, such as the digestive system. Stress and lack of rest also affect us here, the digestive system is strongly controlled by biological rhythms and activity patterns, and not just by what, and when we eat. This means that when those patterns are disrupted the digestive system may find itself with plenty of corrosive acids and enzymes and no food. This can lead to indigestion, heartburn, irritable bowel syndrome (IBS) and ulcers.

Breathing problems can play havoc with the digestive system; problems with snoring and sleep apnoea can cause air to be sucked into the stomach and intestines, which can cause Gastro-oesophageal reflux. (see page 91)

Pain

For various people, pain, a feeling of discomfort, distress, or agony, can make the nighttime intolerable. Even secondary pain or discomfort, like earache, can interfere with good sleep. Protracted and periodic pain is one of the most important causes of sleeping problems and insomnia. An aching back, a sore throat, a headache or migraine, or the pain of a more serious medical condition can all keep your awake at night.

If pain associated with illness disrupts sleep, it does so at the time when the body needs it most. Pain tells us when something is wrong, it is a message and symptom that something we are doing is injuring us, and we had better find out what it is and stop it before serious damage is done. Pain can be malignant and destructive, some are plagued with pain with no obvious cause, amputees can suffer from 'phantom limb pain', with pain coming from a limb they no longer possess. Many more people's lives are made wretched by chronic pain that could be from arthritis, bad backs or sciatica. It is very important to think about your sleeping posture and the comfort and firmness of your bed. Nighttime is often difficult for people with pain and you may be helped considerably by starting off the night on the correct type of bed and mattress and in a posture that is suitable for your condition. If your problem involves neck and head pain, then you should not use high pillows, which raise the head and put a strain on the muscles at the back of the neck.

Keeping your head elevated above the rest of your body while sleeping or laying down will help with pain relief in the lower body and also prevents the regurgitation of acid back up into the esophagus. This can be done by placing bricks under your headboard or by sleeping in an adjustable or hydraulic bed since pillows are not sufficient to relieve night distress. People with back troubles are often better off lying on their backs, but lying on one side with the upper leg drawn up at the knee and supported by a pillow can help leg or hip problems. A disturbed sleep pattern is a major problem for chronic pain suffers, many people say that they have disturbed nights because of pain and as a result feel exhausted and find that they have an overwhelming desire to sleep during the day.

The sleep disturbance usually comes about as a result of tension being present in the body at the time of going to sleep. An exhausted, tense body offers fertile ground for pain to grow and to be reinforced by a stream of negative thoughts and images, which many claim, is their biggest obstacle to sound sleep. You may find it difficult to get off to sleep, wake in the night, or find you are too sleepy to get up in the morning and doze at intervals during the day. This disturbed sleep pattern is common and several factors can be responsible. The severity of the pain may prevent you getting off to sleep, discomfort arising from lying down in one position for too long may wake you up, tension which has built up through the day can be released from knotted, tight muscles during the night and this can cause restlessness and even pain, RLS can sometimes be caused by this. (see page 46)

Getting into bed or waking in the night can often be the signals for a negative stream of thoughts about your health and your seemingly hopeless situation to be switched on, these can produce tension and increase pain. Frustration and anger at your inability to sleep can produce further tension. In this situation sleeplessness can become a habit, it is likely that you go to bed expecting to have difficulty getting off to sleep and that you will wake up during the night because you always do. These expectations can be worrying and it is quite likely that you will live up to them having programmed yourself to a pattern of behaviour which is hindering your attempts to manage pain, and thus get the restful sleep that you need in your life. Now is the time to work on changing this unhelpful pattern and many of the techniques described in this book for managing sleeplessness will also help patients come to terms with pain, i.e. meditation, affirmations, relaxations techniques, massage and complementary therapies such as herbalism, acupuncture, and Chinese medicine.

The Elderly and Infirm

The increase in the number of people over 65 in the 21st century and the rise in the proportion of older people to younger will represent a marked change in the demographic patterns in the world, that will have profound social, economic, medical, and personal consequences. Early in life, most people fall asleep quickly and sleep soundly. As they grow older, they may find settling down to sleep more difficult. They may awaken more often and then take longer to go back to sleep.

A large proportion of older people are at risk from disturbances to sleep that may be caused by many factors such as retirement and changes in social patterns. The demise of spouse and close friends, living alone, increased use of medications, and ongoing diseases. Other contributory lifestyle changes include generally reduced physical activity and more frequent napping. In practical terms, this all means that elderly people have reduced total amounts of daily sleep and are also more easily awakened from sleep at night. In addition, most people over 65 wake up at least once a night for a trip to the bathroom.

While changes in sleep patterns have been viewed as part of the normal aging process, many of these disturbances may be related to pathological processes that are associated with aging. During aging there are typical changes in the pattern of sleep, older people tend to nap and the amount of time spent in the deeper levels of sleep diminishes. There is an associated increase in awakening during sleep and in the total amount of time awake during the night, in part; these changes appear to represent a loss of sleeping hours. Elderly people should try not to nap during the day, better to do something active if you can, read, talk to someone or go for a short walk in the fresh air, if able. Older people may also suffer from a variety of medical and psycho-social problems and these are very often associated with disturbances of sleep.

These may include psychiatric illnesses, particularly depression, Alzheimer's disease, cardiovascular disease, pulmonary disease, arthritis, pain syndrome and many other diseases.

Some drugs such as steroids, Parkinson's disease drugs and some beta-blockers may prevent or disturb sleep. Other drugs, including antihistamines, antidepressants and certain hypotensives, may cause sedation and interfere with normal sleep patterns. Over the counter medications must always be borne in mind, caffeine and alcohol in the evening should be avoided. Situational disturbance, will upset the elderly, these include admission to hospital, moving from one home to another, moving from home to institutional care, or bereavement. Loneliness in these situations is common, and may lead to waking on minimal stimuli, such as slight noise. Difficulty falling asleep, sleep disruption and waking up too early in the morning can be caused by depression, which becomes more common as we grow older.

For some people despondency begins gradually and develops until, feeling blue, becomes a chronic way of life. Others focus on their poor sleep and become convinced that their lives would be better if they could just get a decent night's sleep. As poor sleep patterns develop, some people may stop eating regularly and may lose their usual interest and enjoyment in the activities of daily life. Loss of a loved one often triggers insomnia and depression in the elderly, investigations by Help the Aged have shown that nearly three quarters of newly widowed people report trouble sleeping a month after the death of the partner. One year later, half report that their sleep problems continue. Also many people suffer snoring; sleep apnoea, or periodic movements in sleep (Restless leg syndrome) that can be disruptive to them themselves and to partners. General measures that can be taken are the same as for everybody else, outlined in this book, but it is a good idea to keep active, inactivity is a strong predisposing factor in insomnia. Advanced sleep phase syndrome is the tendency to be 'early to bed and early to rise', which often develops as we grow older. Many people adapt successfully, but some people find that their bodies are ready for bed earlier than they desire, often well before 9 p.m. The physically and mentally alert tend to be less afflicted with sleeping problems, so anything that encourages more physical and mental activity will tend to improve sleep quality. Once retired from work, find a hobby or pastime to keep you busy, join a social club, gym, walk in the open air every day, and be mobile as long as you can.

Do some regular exercise. Tai Ch'i is ideal for older people, (look at my ten point exercise plan in Appendix 3) it was designed for the less mobile, infirm and even wheelchair bound person who still wants to stay flexible. Too often elderly people do not get physically or mentally tired during the day, this will lead to restless nights because they will not be sufficiently tired. Many elderly people go to bed because they are bored or cold or just have always gone to bed early. Most elderly people crave company and fear boredom, in the UK and the USA it is now unusual for the elderly parent to remain in the family home, and take an active role in their children and their grandchildren's lives.

If you are on medications consult your doctor for the best times of day to take them, some prescribed drugs have a stimulating effect, and it would be best for them not to be taken in the evening. Where possible keep your brain stimulated during the daytime as much as possible, even it you can't get out and about the way you used to. Some elderly people, especially those with Alzheimer's disease or other forms of dementia, are susceptible to night wandering. Night wandering is not sleepwalking, those affected are awake, they have short-term memory loss and they become confused as to where they are or what time it is. A change of environment can be a trigger, a new home, new room or any change of scenery can lead to confusion and disorientation. Many elderly people feel alone and unwanted, families don't always have time to come round to visit, and many old people are put into homes were they feel isolated and forgotten. Indeed years ago unwanted old people were put into mental hospital were they often remained until they died. If you are able, try each week to spend some time with an elderly or disabled neighbour or relative. See if they are OK; if they need anything or if they want company just have a chat for half an hour now and again. You can find that people of all ages and circumstances have a lot to offer and it could be a mutually beneficial exchange.

Dementía and Alzheímer's Dísease

Originally classified as a mental disorder involving loss of intelligence, as opposed to amentia, where intelligence is retarded from birth. Thus dementia praecox, premature dementia, now known as schizophrenia. Dementia is now generally taken to mean mental deterioration as a result of physical changes in the brain. Although dementia is often an irreversible manifestation of old age, its symptoms, (loss of memory, concentration, apathy, insomnia, hallucinations and other symptoms more suggestive of psychosis), should not be accepted without further enquiry as some dementia may be helped by treatment. The herb Ginkgo Biloba has proved to be very helpful in cases of dementia. There has also been a lot of research done recently about the effects of selenium (selenium L-Methionine) and it helps prevent cancer and the ageing process. People with dementia are often afraid of the dark and that makes them confused at night, restless and noisy. Treatment with full spectrum light has been known to help many sufferers of night confusion. (see pages 208-209 and appendix 1 for info on full spectrum light)

It is a characteristic of the nervous system that lost brain cells cannot regenerate, and characteristic of all tissues that cells do not last forever. The commonest type of physical change is seen in Alzheimer's disease, where nerve tissue throughout the brain withers and dies. This is an uncommon disease, but similar changes in older people are common and can count for many if not most cases of senile dementia. A much rarer condition, Pick's disease, also affects younger people; the changes affect mainly the frontal lobes of the brain. People with all these conditions tend to sleep badly, they become restless and disorientated, and sometime wander off or talk in their sleep.

Restless Legs Syndrome (RLS) and Periodic Limb Movement Disorder (PLMD).

Everyone experiences muscle cramps from time to time, you may have been sitting too long, walking for a long time or in different shoes. About 15 per cent of healthy people, and as many as 30 per cent of patients with rheumatic arthritis suffer from RLS.

Nocturnal legs cramps can be annoying and painful but someone suffering from restless legs syndrome (RLS) often feel as if they need to move their legs and can't get comfortable. There is often a constrained creeping and crawling feeling or pins and needles deep within the legs or running up and down the legs. This sensation occurs while awake, usually in the evening at bedtime, or during sleep. The movement needed to relieve this feeling may have to be quite vigorous and uncomfortable. Individuals suffering from RLS often also suffer from periodic limb movement disorder (PLMD), but not vice versa. Addiction to caffeine and anaemia can be causes of leg discomfort. If you are post-menopausal, pregnant, trying to lose weight, or don't consume enough calcium, you are vulnerable to developing leg cramps. Iron deficiency can contribute to RLS and too much tea, which contains caffeine, hinders iron absorption in the body.

Periodic-limb-movement disorder usually affects the legs, the movement occur every 15-40 seconds and can be grouped into runs of half a minute to an hour. Bed partners may report kicking and restless movements in their partner's sleep. People with sleep apnoea may move their limbs in their sleep as they struggle for breath. But the cause is often unknown; it may be connected with poor circulation, lack of calcium or other nutrients including Vitamin E, magnesium, potassium , manganese and vitamin A. In women it may be related to hormone levels, and it is often worse when the sufferer is under stress or malnourished in some way.

One thing to try is improving your circulation by taking a footbath in alternate hot and cold water during the evening. Keep the temperature in your bedroom constant if possible, have a free flow of air in the room, or air the room well during the day and don't have heavy or restricting bed covers or night clothes. Because it is known that sugar and caffeine reduce the absorption of vitamins and minerals, particularly calcium, I would advise the elimination of sugar and caffeine from you diet. Smoking decreases the absorption of nutrients from food and should be avoided; including passive smoking. Taking calcium 1200mg at bedtime will help leg cramps and to promote healthy sleep, try Dolomite tablets, vitamin E and fish oil supplements in capsule form. Regular exercise will also help by keeping the joints supple and less likely to cramp, but you must take care in warming up and cooling down before and after exercise, and building up slowly and not trying to undertake too much too soon.

Cramps and Night Cramps
Cramp is a prolonged, painful and involuntary contraction of a muscle any muscle can be affected, these spasms can commonly occur during the night most commonly in the calf or the foot. The best way to alleviate the problem is with massage and stretching, however, nutrition is the most

effective long-term solution. Eating foods high in vitamin E may help improve the poor circulation that can cause night cramps. Night cramps in the elderly may also be helped by vitamin B12, found in foods such as fish, eggs, cheese and pork.

Tinnitus

From the Latin 'tinnere' tinnitus describes the condition of noises heard 'in the ear or ears' and/or 'in the head'. Tinnitus is an incessant noise, buzzing, or ringing in the inner ear that makes it difficult to relax and hard to fall asleep. About 40 per cent of adults can experience tinnitus at one time or another in their lives. Some 10 per cent suffer from chronic tinnitus, stress and insomnia is linked to tinnitus and it can be brought on by stressful situations. Many sufferers say that tinnitus affects their ability to get to sleep and interferes with the quality of their sleep, waking them up and leaving them debilitated and tired the next day.

It seems most likely that tinnitus does not actually wake people, but of course, it can be the first thing they notice when a natural awakening occurs. It also seems that more women are likely to have sleep disturbances due to tinnitus than men but the reasons for this are not obvious. The cause of chronic tinnitus is usually unclear, it could be caused by wax in the ear-hole, blockage of the eustachian tube with common cold, and irritation of the auditory nerve could cause it. Tinnitus noises have no external source; they are described variously as ringing, whistling, buzzing and humming, amongst other things. Many people experience two or more different noises at once, either continuously, or interrupted by periods of silence. Tinnitus has many common consequences, and these include insomnia and depression. In the night even mild tinnitus can seem deafening, as a result tinnitus undermines the concentration and leaves you tired and irritable. Leaving the radio on very low can help, or listening to music on headphones dulls the buzzing of tinnitus. You can get a pad linked to a radio, CD player or tape-cassette player and this seems to help tinnitus suffers by blocking out the sound of the tinnitus and enabling one to sleep. For more information about tinnitus and about pillow maskers and pillow speakers contact the British Tinnitus Association tel 0114 279 6600)

Migraine

About six million people in the UK suffer from migraine, for some it is a headache that they can put up with, but for many others, migraine is a devastating attack on work, family and social life. Migraine is a common and distressing kind of headache, sometimes with no evident cause. Attacks can last a few hours and are often brought on by stress or bright lights. Warning symptoms such as a sense of flickering lights before the eyes are common, during the attack the patient cannot stand bright light. Most patients feel nauseated during or after the attack, and some people do actually vomit.

The site of the trouble seems to be the arteries inside and outside the skull, they constrict, restricting blood to the brain. It is thought that migraine is caused by changes to chemicals and blood vessels in the brain, but why this happens is still unknown. A migraine is typically a throbbing pain, usually located on one side of the head. Other symptoms may include visual disturbance, feeling or being sick and sensitivity to light, sound and smells.

As migraine is often associated with stress, regular massage, reflexology or Indian head massage which will release a lot of the tension in the body.

Migraine and headaches can severely disturb sleep; if you get one as you go to bed it can disturb getting to sleep. After a migraine the person can often fall into very heavy sleep and can awake sometimes feeling heavy and listless. If you do suffer from headache it is important that you avoid the trigger factors causing the headaches and help lessen the pain and discomfort once it has started. Before you can do much, though, it is important to have some idea of what is causing your headache. With so many different possibilities, from eye strain, sleep apnoea, high blood pressure, sinus problems, allergies, eating ice-cream to tension, it is not surprising that there is no one common treatment that works for all headaches. Treatments vary according to the cause discover what is provoking your headache or migraine and then you have a good chance of avoiding them.

If you also suffer from neck and back problems it may be advisable to see a specialist chiropractor, osteopath or massage therapist. Keeping a diary can help record foods you may have eaten, alcohol and events or situations that caused tension.

Also record what measures you took, pills, hot or cold compress, massage, etc. and how effective the treatment was. Stress is the main cause of most headaches, and environmental conditions like stuffy rooms, pollution, bad smells, light and temperature are the main contenders for many other headache and migraines. Fresh air is the enemy of headaches, walk in the fresh air everyday and take regular exercise. The practice of stress relieving techniques like meditation, deep breathing exercises, yoga and Tai Chi are also very helpful. There are many herbal remedies, homeopathic remedies and supplements that can help, I find Ginkgo Biloba very helpful, Ginkgo Biloba helps blood transport oxygen and other vital nutrients to the brain, and other extremities of the body, such as the hands and feet. It can help relieve headaches, migraine, tinnitus, memory loss, and slow down the aging process and dementia. (See appendix 1 for useful addresses for further help with headaches and migraine)

Sleep Headaches

Sleeping too long, too deeply, too little, or having interrupted sleep may all give rise to headaches and migraines. A hot stuffy room or sleeping in a draught can also bring on headaches. Even if the mechanism is in doubt there are some obvious answers.

About fifteen per cent of people develop a headache if they do not get up at their normal time. If this happens to you, it does not mean that you can never sleep in, but you will have to experiment on how much time you can sleep in without getting a headache. This explains why some people who don't have the opportunity to sleep well during the week wake up with a headache at the weekend. One reason for this could be that many people relax more at the weekend, maybe drink more alcohol, which increases depth and duration of sleep, and may also cause migraine or headache.

Many years ago 'sleep rationing' was tried as a treatment for migraine, with some success. Heavy food, drugs, alcohol, caffeine and too little physical exercise, can all lead to a longer lie in and heavy head as a result. Avoid smoky atmospheres and never sleep in a smoke polluted room. Headaches due to insufficient or interrupted sleep have previously been confused with tension headaches and attributed to psychological upset. Recently, however, they have been recognised as something different. Unlike tension headaches, the headache of sleep deprivation responds well to simple treatment like having a short nap or a walk in the fresh air.

Epilepsy

An epileptic fit is an episode of disorganized and excessive activity in a part of the brain, causing disturbances of sensation, movement, or consciousness according to the area of the brain that is involved. With petit mal epilepsy the only symptom is fleeting loss of consciousness. The stronger grand mal is the type of fit in which the patient sometimes falls unconscious often with a cry, the muscles stiffen and then twitch violently, often the person will bite his tongue and the bladder may empty, the attack can last a couple of minutes. Epilepsy can be very distressing both for the individual with the condition and for the friends and family. Often the cause is not clear and this can make it difficult to treat.

Fits can be caused by a variety of factors, and in well over half of the cases the cause remains unknown. A very high proportion of people will have at least one convulsion in their life, usually when ill and in early childhood. Stress plays a major part in epilepsy. Something may be worrying you or and lack of sleep and general debility can also play a part. The first recommendations given to those with epilepsy are those given to most people for a healthy life. To try to make your life as stable as possible, by eating regular meals and keeping to regular sleeping hours. Take regular, but not excessive exercise, eat properly and keep stress to a minimum. Epilepsy attacks while one is asleep are not uncommon and can be very distressful for all concerned, but modern medicine does reduce the frequency of attacks.

Chapter 8

Skin Complaints and Allergies

Skin conditions in themselves are not sleep disorders, but they can impede your slumber, make you uncomfortable and cause very restless sleep that if combined with other problems could lead to insomnia. Insect bites and skin parasites can be a problem at night when they often feel hot and itchy keeping you awake from scratching and general discomfort and bedsores will make life intolerable for those confined to bed if they are not careful. Children can suffer from nappy rash, and people of all ages can get allergic reactions and heat rashes, all of which can make for a recipe for restless nights. It is important to keep cool, as heat aggravates most skin complaints, for instance eczema, psoriasis and dermatitis. Avoid synthetic materials, and take care of soaps, detergents, cosmetics, animals, and material fibres like wool that may cause irritation or allergic reaction. Get medical advice and don't delay getting treatment for any unusual rash or irritation, it may be harmless but it may also be contagious so act quickly to avoid passing on any infection to others.

Dermatitis

In its literal sense (inflammation of the skin) this term might mean almost any skin disease, but in practice it is applied to inflammation confined to the skin, with itch, vesicles or bullae (small or large blisters) that may exude fluid, and formation of scales. Inflammations due to infection by viruses, bacteria or fungi (e.g. herpes, impetigo, ringworm) are not included. Irritants such as solvents, chemicals, and detergents may cause contact dermatitis. A metal watch strap or piece of jewellery can also set up a reaction even after there has been contract with the item for a long time, in some cases even years. Some plants will set off a response; poison ivy and primrose are two well-known irritants. One can also occasionally get an allergic reaction or rash if taking an herbal or homeopathic remedy, if you do stop taking it unless undergoing a purge under a therapist's guidance.

Eczema

Eczema is a group of diseases, with inflammation of the skin, itch, and blisters that may seep fluid and scale the skin. The term eczema applies to disorders that were thought to be inherent rather than due to contact with particular agents. There are different kinds of eczema the kind of eczema most talked about is called 'contact' eczema. It is now recognised that many substances will cause an eczematous reaction such substances include detergents. Nappy rash appears to be just such a reaction of young and sensitive skin to urine and faeces. Some variations are as follows:

• Atopic eczema, which means practically the same as allergic eczema, is often associated with allergic conditions such as hay fever and asthma. It commonly starts in infancy, and although as a rule it clears up before puberty it some times persists into adult life or reoccurs at times of stress.

• Seborrhoeic eczema, usually confines itself to the scalp with the formation and shedding of greasy scales (dandruff). In only a few severe cases it spreads to the eyebrows, sides of the nose, ears and front of the chest.

• Nummular (discoid) eczema, affects middle-aged or elderly people, men more than women. The typical lesions are reddish discs 1-2 cm across, in limbs and trunk. It can appear suddenly and disappear just as quickly, it is thought to be brought on by stress or upsetting situations.

• Varicose eczema, more correctly hypostatic or stasis eczema is a mild inflammation and scaling with brown discoloration of the skin of the lower legs, and ankles. Can be caused by poor circulation and inactivity.

• Lichen simplex, appears as patches of thickened, sometimes pigmented skin. The condition causes itching and is brought on by emotional stress.

Psoriasis

A common disorder of the outer layer of the skin, the appearance is of thickened red blotches and a scaly surface, most often on the scalp, back, and arms. Psoriasis can be brought on by trauma or stress and it common among people suffering emotional strain. It can also be connected with general poor health and with rheumatism and arthritis. Psoriasis greatly benefits from natural sunlight and fresh air. Application of avocado oil is very soothing for eczema and psoriasis and camomile and lavender essential oils can help some people if used in very small dilution for application or massage. These oils are also very calming and will help in preparation for sleep.

Impetigo

Impetigo is an infection of the outer layers of the skin by aphylococci, forming clusters of small abscesses. It is highly contagious, especially among children and from the original site other areas of the persons own skin can be infected by contact.

Herpes

Two distinct virus infections, herpes simplex and herpes zoster, both cause clusters of sore blisters on the skin, and both, once established, lie dormant waiting to erupt. Herpes simplex involves two types of infection caused by slightly different strains of the virus. Type 1, cold sores on lips, nose and face, and type 2 on the sexual organs that is transmitted sexually. Herpes zoster (shingles) is caused by the virus of chickenpox, the virus may lurk un-noticed for many years, and then, emerge at times of stress.

Ringworm

Ringworm is one of the commonest skin diseases; it is an infection of the outer layer of the skin and is caused by a microscopical fungus or mould. The most common sites are the scalp, the groin and between the toes. Itching is common to all forms. With ringworm of the scalp, small patches of hair are temporarily lost. The nails of the fingers or toes may harbour the fungus and become deformed, often in association with athlete's foot.

Athlete's foot

Athlete's foot is ringworm of the feet and infection of the skin with a fungus especially, between the outer toes. The only association with athletics is that the changing rooms of schools and sports clubs are likely places for the infection to be passed on.

Hay fever, allergic rhinitis

For some, insomnia is a more seasonal problem. They are fine during the winter months, but come the spring the dreadful combination of streaming eyes, a blocked nose and cough makes their life and their bed a most uncomfortable place and peaceful sleep hard to achieve. April, May, June, July and

August can be malevolent months for the many thousands of hay fever sufferers in Britain and in many other parts of the world. And it seems that there are more sufferers around now than ever before. The number of allergic disorders is doubling every ten years. Hay fever is actually the common name for an allergic reaction to an airborne substance. Usually the substance is pollen but it can be a fungus, mold, mildew, dust mites, pet fur or cockroaches.

High pollen counts, pollution, global warming, longer and warmer summers are all possible culprits. If helps it you know what kind of pollen or pollution is causing your particular problem, you can then attempt to avoid it. Tree pollens are the first to arrive, starting as early as April, the grass pollens, which are the worst offenders peak in June and July, while shrub pollens have a longer season. (You can get more information from National Pollen Research Unit)

The drug Piriton is often prescribed for allergic reactions and conditions, it has the side effect of helping to aid restful sleep. Piriton should not be given to young children and should not be used for long periods of time, as it will cause drowsiness, impaired reactions and dizziness. There are many antihistamines that are often prescribed to relieve itching, sneezing and hay fever. The most troublesome side effect is sedation and lethargy, which is common, but they can also cause dry mouth, blurring of vision, and constipation. Some research has shown that large doses of vitamin C and B6, together with the minerals zinc and calcium, have a protective effect, as does evening primrose oil. Hay fever or allergic rhinitis sufferers will also be affected and their symptoms made worse by cigarette smoke, fur and feathers, house dust and traffic fumes.

Using eye pads, with rosewater or camomile infusions, not the essential oils themselves but the liquid that is left over when essential oils are distilled, can cool eyes.

Burners with a few drops of camomile, eucalyptus or lavender can also be very calming, also use in a steam inhalation or a drop or two on a hankie or tissue to sniff whenever needed during the day.

Asthma

The original meaning of asthma is heavy breathing or difficulty breathing, but now the word is taken to mean a particular kind of difficulty arising from spasm of involuntary muscle around the small branches of the air tubes in the lungs.

Allergies can contribute to snoring by causing swelling of the mucous membranes of the mouth, throat and airways they can also cause asthma. If a poor sleeper is known to have allergies, or has asthma, hay fever, conjunctivitis or contact dermatitis, the role of allergens is causing the sleeping problem and should always be investigated. The cause can be common allergens like pollen, animal fur or feathers, the house dust mite, cigarette smoke, or other pollution agents.

Dust mites are invisible to the naked eye, this tiny insect can cause allergies and asthma, and they thrive in warm, moist conditions, like beds, but also carpets, curtains and soft toys. It is not the actual mite but its droppings that cause the problem; many experts believe that dust mites cause 50 per cent of asthma cases. It you have problem with asthma and or allergies, vacuum all bedroom furnishings regularly, and consider getting rid of the bedroom carpet in favour of a wooden, cork, vinyl or alternative floor covering and blinds instead of curtains. Wash bed linen regularly at a high temperature and buy pillows with anti-allergy covers to keep the mites away. Mites love humidity, a good dehumidifier will kill them off, and in the long-term can decrease asthma attacks, and improve sleep. There are anti-mite sprays, but their effects are only temporary.

Always sleep in a well aired room, not too hot or too cold, if agents in the outside world, pollens, are causing the problem you could consider using a fan in hot weather or fine mesh or netting over open windows. It is advisable to drink plenty of fluids, and a warm drink like herbal teas tend to help asthma suffers. Avoid very cold or very hot air, and try to prevent colds developing. Take a good multivitamin and mineral supplement and eat a healthy diet, full of whole foods, fruit and vegetables.

Allergies

There are more people with food allergies than we realize, and it is the most common undiagnosed health problem today. Ailments like respiratory problems, Irritable Bowel Syndrome, and depression are often caused by food allergies.
Why have food allergies become so common in today's world? There is greater stress on our immune system caused by pollution, in a world were there are more food choice that every before, why are more people eating a limited or inadequate diet? More mothers are using bottle feeds instead of breast-feeding and our food sources are adulterated, genetically altered and full of additives. Some of the most common food allergies are dairy products, wheat products, peanuts, but it could be anything.

Not only food and drink also water, the atmosphere, dust and furnishings, can cause the disturbances and allergies that are often associated with insomnia, depression, anxiety, skin complaints, digestive complaints as well as many other physical symptoms.

Allergens, or allergy provoking particles, can consist of any substance found in the environment or in our food, which the body regards as alien and potentially harmful to our body. Our immune system responds with an armoury of antibodies released into the bloodstream or tissues. Individual reactions vary from sniffles and sneezes to the potentially fatal reaction suffered by people who are allergic to peanuts or bee stings. Allergy related illnesses seem to be increasing rapidly; one in three children now exhibit symptoms of asthma, eczema or hay fever before the age of eleven.

Testing for allergies can be a lengthy process, one of slowly eliminating certain items for a period of one or two weeks and then evaluating the differences in your health. It is a good idea to keep a food diary and record any digestive, skin, sleep or mood effects. There are allergy-testing kits available kinsiology can also be very helpful in discovering food and other substance intolerance, by testing the muscles reactions to different items.

Chapter 9

Digestion and Digestive Problems

Even before you have taken the first taste of any food, its aroma trigger's the digestive system. An efficient digestive system is vital for good health, without it, vitamins, minerals, trace elements, fats, the body cannot absorb proteins and carbohydrates. Indigestion is often the result of eating large meals quickly or late at night. If you suffer from indigestion at night, try spreading you're eating more evenly through the day and having the larger meals early in the day, rather than later.

Cut down on fatty foods with stimulate the output of acid in the gut. Too much alcohol also increases stomach acidity. Constipation, flatulence and bad breath, are often caused by fermented fibre, and can also result for poor eating habits, repeated attacks of severe pain may be a sign of gallstones. A bloated abdomen or pain, especially in the low left side of the abdomen, accompanied by wind and alternating diarrhoea and constipation, may be a sign of Irritable Bowel Syndrome. Long-term alcohol abuse can result in gastritis and ulcers. Colitis and Crohn's disease reduce the amount of nutrients absorbed during digestion.

The Irritable Bowel Syndrome (IBS)

Irritable bowel syndrome, also known as spastic colon or nervous indigestion is a common and frustrating problem. In simple terms, IBS is a condition in which the large intestine fails to function as it should. Normally, regular muscular contractions of the large intestine move waste from the small intestine to the rectum at which point it's evacuated. But when IBS is present, excessive muscular contractions of the large intestine result in cramping and diarrhoea, and the lack of contractions results in constipation and cramping. The most common effecting foods include dairy products, grains and wheat products. Caffeine can also cause problems, because it is a bowel stimulant as are many artificial sweeteners. Nicotine, like caffeine, can cause bowel disturbances. If you smoke, it could be affecting your symptoms and you really should quit. Many studies show that psychological disturbances play a role in IBS. Some studies have shown that people with IBS have higher levels of anxiety than normal and also a greater tendency to depression.

Many sufferers of IBS complain of insomnia although rarely is it due to actual pain. Many say they are aware of wind but it does not really cause discomfort, only a feeling of extreme wakefulness. Although many IBS sufferers have food allergies or do not drink sufficient water, between 1 and 2 litres per day, they may also not eat regularly, sensibly, they may have poor bacteria in the gut or they may eat too late in the evening. It is accepted that food allergy symptoms are much worse if you are hot; so one recommendation is a cool shower before retiring to bed. It is also know that bacteria in the gut produces chemicals, which make us sleepy, so if there is an imbalance in the gut flora this effect may be reduced. Natural live yoghurt is good for restoring intestinal balance and you could try Yackult, which is very good for restoring the intestinal bacteria naturally. (Food combining can help some IBS suffers see pages 242-243 also see useful addresses in appendix 1for more information about IBS)

Blood Sugar

One lesser-known cause of sleeplessness is low blood sugar, if you wake up in the early hours thirsty or craving something sweet it could be because your blood sugar has dropped. It may be that you ate a meal at 6 pm and your blood sugar levels dropped over the evening. Try eating a banana or one sweet biscuit with a glass of water or milk before going to bed. If you experience regular loss of energy, excessive urination and thirst for no apparent reason it would be advisable to get your GP to check for diabetes. (see page 94 for more information on diabetes)

It is also very important not to de-hydrate over night always have a small drink at bed time, but not too much so that you wake up wanting to go to the loo.

Circulation Problems

There are three main factors that cause circulation problems, including heart disease, smoking, high blood pressure and high blood cholesterol levels.

Obesity can lead to the last two and drinking alcohol to excess is also a major cause of high blood pressure. However, as we get older many people who are not overweight and do not smoke or drink still develop high blood pressure and high blood cholesterol levels.

Related circulatory problems are chest pains at times of stress, diabetes sufferers are particularly prone to circulatory disorders as thickening of the walls of the arteries is a known complication of the disease. Two other circulation problems that affect the extremities include Raynaud's disease and chilblains.

In Raynaud's disease, the fingers or toes become white and numb when cold and when warmed tingle painfully as the blood returns. Chilblains usually result from exposure to cold, but they can be a problem at normal temperatures when people have poor circulation. They usually occur in fingers and toes, but they can also affect ears, cheeks and the nose. A severe itching and burning sensation that results from insufficient blood in the affected area. The herb Ginkgo Biloba can be of great help in circulatory problems, as can partaking in some regular exercise. If cold feet are a problem in bed wear some socks, but don't fall into the error of having too many bedclothes or heavy blankets, light covers that don't weigh down on you too heavily, such as continental quilts, are best, as long as you are warm.

Cirrhosis

Damage caused by cirrhosis, cannot easily be repaired, cirrhosis is caused by alcohol, which, will have affected the body's ability to absorb and store life sustaining vitamins and minerals. The patient will lose weight, not be able sleep, and have to eliminate alcohol and be very careful with their diet on a long road to recovery. The most common cause of cirrhosis is alcohol abuse; other causes include viral hepatitis, malnutrition, and chronic inflammation or blockage of ducts in liver. Alcohol and particularly over use of alcohol and sleep problems are often intrinsically linked as mentioned in Chapter 6.

Anorexia

The word anorexia means loss of appetite, however, loss of appetite in the sense of never being hungry is not a central or necessary feature of anorexia nervosa. In fact, an anorexic may at times be very hungry. Anorexia is more about weight than about eating, the central feature of the disorder is a body weight, which is abnormally low for the age, height and sex of the person. The anorexic has a phobia or a morbid fear or avoidance of her/his normal body weight.

Anorexia nervosa is a serious illness of which almost the only symptom is that the patient either refuses to eat food or, will under protest, eat and then secretly vomit everything up again. This in time leads to under-nourishment, starvation, and occasionally death. The three central features of anorexia nervosa are an abnormally low body weight; an attitude and behaviour, which tends to maintain this low weight (weight phobia) and other occurrences such as (amenorhoea), the absence of menstrual periods, which is a frequent consequence of this illness. Of course, anorexia nervosa with weight phobia is not the only psychiatric state, which may lead people to lose weight and eat oddly. Psychotic disorder with delusions about contamination of foods, depression of mood with true loss of appetite, obsession states and interpersonal difficulties with those who are involved in providing food, may all lead to states which closely resemble true anorexia nervosa, but the weight phobia will be absent.

Nearly all the patients are adolescent or young adult girls; more rarely does it affect boys or older people although there are now more cases among other groups including young children. The sleep of the anorexic subject is usually disturbed and she/he will tend to wake early or be disturbed more easily. Anorexia nervosa is evidently a severe neurosis in which unconscious refusal to accept puberty and adult sexuality is an important factor. Despite the relaxation of sexual taboos of modern times, this illness appears to be on the increase. This may be partly due to the popular insistence that slender is beautiful and healthy as portrayed in fashion magazines.

Anorexia can also be brought on by stressful situations, unhappy home life, and bullying or physical or sexual abuse. The patient will usually insist that she/he eats enough and any more would make them fat, and is often accompanied by over strenuous exercise and sometimes self mutilation.

Serious long term weight loss lowers body temperature and has a damaging effect on sleep, anorexics often have digestive problems, may cease to have periods, feelings of stress and depression and low worth, which will all contribute to sleepless nights and an agitated state during the day.

Bulimia

Bulimia is compulsive over eating, usually a symptom of emotional disturbance. It is most common in adolescent girls but also affecting other groups of society, including the depressed of any age, the overweight, and young children. Typically the patient follows a burst of over eating by self-induced vomiting or purging and recrimination. For quite often, and despite some appearances, the person may be genuinely worried about putting on weight, even if unable to control eating habits. Bulimia often accompanies anorexia nervosa, binges of mindless gluttony alternating with spells of deliberate starvation. Though on its own bulimia does not carry the risk to health and life of anorexia it is a distressing complaint. Treatment, by highly specialized psychotherapy, may be reinforced by anti-depressant medication. Many complementary therapies have been proved to help bulimia and anorexia dramatically in conjunction with medical supervision. The main objective is to restore the person's self-esteem massage and reflexology can really help if performed by a trusted friend or therapist.

Insomnia is a common problem brought on by eating disorders like anorexia nervosa and bulimia. It can be caused by the underlying stress and depression that cause the disease. And by the very physical discomfort brought about by the condition of the person's body, i.e. stomach cramps, over thinness and bony body, aching joints and muscles from over exercise and being unable to get comfortable generally in bed.

Obesity

Obesity is an unhealthy excess of body weight, surplus weight puts a burden on the body by imposing an unnecessary weight on joints and muscles. The heart has not only to work harder, but its efficiency suffers from fat deposited in its muscle. The chances of developing diabetes and hypertension are also increased.

Ideal weight varies according to sex, bone structure and metabolism. Some people have heavier frames and some carry more muscle than others. The crucial factor is the amount of fat, and especially the fat belly, women tend to collect fat deposits around the thighs and buttocks and men around their middles and will develop large tummies.

Some theories suggest that the mechanisms of the body set a threshold at which weight remains steady, and that fat people overeat because the threshold is somehow advanced.

Heredity plays an important part; fat parents tend to breed fat children, partly by their example and partly by inherited eating habits.

Environmental factors other then upbringing include social pressures; people that overeat also tend to over drink. Overweight people and those that are heavy drinkers tend to have more problems with breathing during sleep, such as snoring and apnoea. Extreme over weight can cause sleeplessness and restless nights, a heavy body can find it difficult to get comfortable may have more digestive problems and can have aches and pains in limbs from the strain of carrying a heavy body. Being overweight can cause

Gastro-oesophageal Reflux, Heartburn

Gastro-oestophageal reflux is the back up of stomach contents into the esophagus (commonly known as heartburn, because of the pain or tightness it generates in the chest area) can awaken a person various times a night.

Gastro-oesophageal reflux occurs when acid escapes from the stomach and comes back up towards the mouth. On the way it burns the delicate tissues of the oesophagus, causing heartburn. It may stimulate nerves, causing coughing, or reach the entrance to the lungs causing choking, if it reaches the mouth, you may vomit.

When reflux occurs during the day, a few swallows and a vertical position will usually clear the irritating materials from the esophagus. But during sleep, less frequent swallowing and a lying down position can lead reflux to result in waking up coughing and choking. Elevation of the head of the bed on 6 to 8 bricks can help if reflux is a particular problem. This gentle slope will reduce the rate and severity of reflux, pillow or wedges are less effective, and may even make the condition worse because of the way they bend your body at the waist.

Avoid eating large meals within three hours of bedtime and avoid foods and beverages that particularly stimulate your stomach. These may include spicy or greasy foods, coffee, chocolate, and beer. Get more exercise, fitter people and people near to their ideal weight generally have less digestive problems.

Avoid cigarette smoke during a meal, eating standing up or with a plate on your lap in front of the television. If you possibly can sit at a table, allow sufficient time to eat slowly and chew your food well. Don't drink copious amount of fluid with your meal. It is better to drink a glass of water half an hour before a meal especially if you want to lose weight. Stomach aches; indigestion and intestinal problems are one of the prime causes for insomnia and disturbed sleep.

Chapter 10

The Immune System

The immune system is a highly complex and many layered defence mechanism, designed to protect us against the abounding multitudes of micro organisms (bacteria, viruses, parasites) that see us as a potential host. The system's main defences consist of trillions of cells, which circulate through the entire body, always alert and on the lookout for hostile invasion. These cells (lymphocytes) are pumped around the body in the bloodstream, but drain back to the heart via the lymphatics, a system of small vessels rather like veins that drain back through the lymph glands in the neck, groin and under the armpits before emptying back into the bloodstream. These lymphocytes grab hold of any bacteria, virus or infection, they multiply, which is why swollen lymph glands are a sure sign of infection, and they release antibodies.

Not all harmful substances get past these defenders, very little does, but there are some bugs which are so virulent that they seem to be able to break through our defences, or sabotage them. The AIDS virus is a case in point, but there are other areas of potential weakness. Malnutrition, stress, smoking, alcohol and insomnia all weaken our bodies self defence mechanisms, dieting or a restrictive or limited diet will weaken the lymphatic system. Many elderly people have an increased susceptibility to infection, due to a faltering immune system. Doctors used to think that this was an unavoidable aspect of ageing, but with exercise and good nutrition it need not be so. Smoking is definitely a problem, as it hits the immune system hard, and weakens it considerably. Smokers are prone to more diseases and will take longer to shake them off once afflicted. This is why smoking is associated with an increased risk of cancer, not just of the lungs, but also the mouth, larynx, and most other parts of the body. Stress lowers resistance generally, takes away the will to fight infections, disrupt sleep patterns and reduces appetite, all indications of lowered immunity. Insomnia and lack of sleep will certainly impair the function of the body's immune system and weaken resistance to sickness and infections.

HIV and Aids

HIV (human immune deficiency virus), previous know as human T-cell lymphotrophic virus type 111. The virus invades T-lymphocytes, a type of white blood cell on which cellular immunity depends. No cure or vaccine has yet been found for AIDS (Acquired Immune Deficiency Syndrome), although the quality of life of its sufferers may be improved by the right choice of foods, supplementation and drugs. Similarly, people with HIV (Human Immunodeficiency Virus), which eventually, but not inevitably, can lead to full blown AIDS. AIDS is a disease in which the body's immune system breaks down, so patient's bodies are no longer efficient at fighting disease. Signs of the onset of HIV or AIDS are weight loss, general debility and could include insomnia. There may also be swollen glands in the groin, neck and armpits, cold sores and other skin disorders. As the disease progresses, patients may suffer from pneumonia, malnutrition and various cancers.

Diabetes

Diabetes is a disease in which the body cannot properly convert food into energy, either because it does not produce enough insulin, or because the cells have become insulin resistant or incapable of absorbing it. Insulin, which is a hormone produced by the pancreas, to regulate the level of glucose, or blood sugar, in the bloodstream. When the blood glucose rises, the pancreas releases insulin, which promotes the absorption of glucose by the body's tissues, with diabetes this process breaks down.

Diabetes can appear at any age, but it does fall into two main kinds, insulin dependent and non-insulin dependent:

• The first one will affect younger people who feel unwell for a few weeks or months and may become very ill if they do not receive insulin, and they must take insulin injections every day.

• The second will affect older people who may have had diabetes for many years before it was discovered and who do not feel particularly ill. This type is often genetic and will run in families and can be more easily controlled with diet and proper lifestyle management.

Diabetes affects up to 200 million people worldwide, and is increasing, especially in children. It is more common for people of northern European origins, estimates suggest that in Britain, up to one person in fifteen is affected by diabetes, mostly with type 2, but fewer that half of these cases are ever diagnosed and treated. People with diabetes have a much higher rate of heart attacks, strokes, and high blood pressure and cataracts, poor circulation to lower limbs, and problems with legs and feet, it can also bring about loss of sensation, burning, pain, and sexual impotence. Diabetes will affect sleep if the blood glucose becomes unbalanced during the night and disturbs the sleep, this can often be overcome by having a light snack before going to bed. Patients can suffer from sore feet, and loss of sensation and the circulation can become weakened this can also impede getting a sound night's sleep. A good diet and healthy lifestyle is imperative for all diabetics, sound sleep and adequate but controlled exercise is vital to maintain fitness and sugar levels at a constant.

Thyroid Disorders

The thyroid is an endocrine gland in the front of the neck it consists of two lobes, one at either side of the Adam's apple, joined at their lower ends by a bridge of glandular tissue across the upper part of the trachea. The principal hormones of the thyroid are thyroxine and tri-iodothyronine. When released into the circulation they promote the synthesis of proteins throughout the body, and they increase the rate at which oxygen is used to ingest fuel reserves and with it the output of energy.

A second thyroid hormone, calcitonin, regulates the concentration of calcium in the blood, calcium is needed for healthy bones but it is also needed in the blood to help with clotting and for nerves and muscles to work properly.

A under active or over active thyroid gland will upset the bodies balance and sleep clock systems by keeping you awake and over active or making you lethargic and sleepy during the day.

Disorders of the thyroid come in different forms:

• Cretinism is when the gland fails to develop in the newborn. The child's physical and mental development are retarded, the child's appearance is distinguished by coarse hair and skin, protruding tongue and potbelly. If given thyroxine from an early age the child will develop normally.

• Thyroid deficiency starting in adult life causes myxoedema, the patient, often a middle aged woman, loses energy and appetite, slow heart rate, lethargy, the body temperature is low, the skin is dry and puffy, and the mind is dulled.

• Goitre is any enlargement of the thyroid gland, simple goitre arises from lack of iodine in the diet, when the body is deprived of iodine is produces more thyroxine and the thyroid gland gets larger until it protrudes in a large swelling in the neck.

• Toxic goitre symptoms arise from an excess of circulating hyroxine, this condition affects 5 times more women than it does men.

• Hyper secretion in an adult is called Graves disease, this again occurs more often in women and is a disorder of the immune system. The basal metabolic rate (BMR) is raised, causing weight loss, insomnia, feeling hot, fast heart beat and increased sweating. A peculiar symptom is that the eyes protrude.

TATT Tired all the Time

Exhaustion, tiredness, lethargy, some reports suggest that nearly half the population suffer from unexplained exhaustion. You may feel exhausted yourself for no apparent

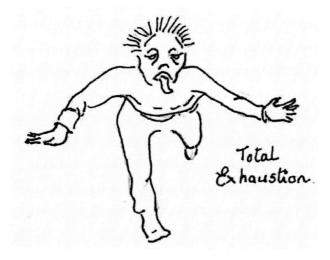

Total Exhaustion.

reason. A new condition has appeared, TATT, tired all the time. There may be some underlying physiological reason, including low blood pressure, hypothyroidism, an under active thyroid gland, and thrytoxicosism and overactive one, anaemia or iron deficiency, rheumatoid arthritis and the debilitating myalgic encephalomyelitis (ME). You need to establish that you are not just tired from overwork, depression, or fluctuating hormones, and that you're not in the recovery period from a viral infection or illness, which could leave you feeling very tired and run down. It is estimated that about 45 per cent of tiredness is caused by psychological or lifestyle reasons which, if they were recognized and dealt with could be resolved. Our working environment, electromagnetic stress, faulty air conditioning, comfort and posture all take a role.

Chapter 11

Pregnancy, Babies, Children and Teenagers

Pregnancy and Childbirth

During the first three months of pregnancy many women are commonly tired and desperate for naps during the day, this can be due to the increased levels of the hormone progesterone in the body. They will also often wake up feeling sick and uncomfortable in the mornings, and as the pregnancy progresses their bodies will feel heavy, unwieldy and it will be more difficult to get comfortable in bed.

In the last few months of pregnancy, with the baby kicking and other discomforts, like having to urinate more frequency, it is often difficult to get a good night's sleep.

A relaxing bath with a few drops of neroli, lavender or marjoram in the later months of pregnancy is very soothing, and you can add ylang ylang for its calming, sedative effect, a maximum of six drops in total for an adult bath. Two drops of rose or lavender on the edge of the pillow will help induce restful sleep.

During pregnancy and especially during the last few months a woman must consult with her doctor if she plans to take any complementary medicines or therapies.

The same thing applies to nursing mothers; the utmost of care must be taken to ensure that you do not pass anything on via milk or bodily contact that may be harmful to the baby. Massage throughout pregnancy is quite safe and very relaxing but once again check with your doctor first. The therapist will only use light techniques and it is fine to gently massage the abdomen, and it often seems to soothe the baby, if the correct oils are used massage will deter stretch marks. An important thing to note if having aromatherapy massage, is that certain essential oils are harmful at some stages of pregnancy, make sure your therapist is aware that you are pregnant and only uses essential oils that are safe at that time. Raising the legs slightly above the head will aid sleep and when the feet are higher than the head it can also help to alleviate swelling and aching in the legs.

Babies also love to be massaged and often find it very relaxing and soothing, it can also help with the bonding process between mother and child.

Babies and Children
The arrival of a new baby is bound to cause a disruption from your normal routine and previous sleep patterns. Parents, who accept that their sleep will be broken, can suffer less from fatigue than those who feel resentful about it.

Be well prepared, if breast feeding, have the baby near to hand for minimal disturbance to sleep, if bottle feeding have everything ready to feed the infant with the least fuss and disruption to all concerned. Breast fed babies will tend to wake more frequently because mother's milk is easily assimilated and after about 3 to 4 hours baby will be ready for more. Breast fed babies can feed in the night without really waking up and are easily put back to bed again. Some babies are difficult to put to sleep and may wake frequently at night for no apparent reason, an homeopathic remedy can often help, but first always check a few basic comforts such as: is the child hot or cold, hungry, ill, anxious about something, or plain just not tired.

Most parents will experience some problems with getting their new baby or young child to sleep soundly through the night at some time or another. In young babies, sleeping problems at night are to be expected, but a baby can quite quickly learn to fall asleep by his/herself. Once an infant or young child begins to associate falling asleep with being rocked or held, they can forget the idea of how to return to sleep on their own. If a child is picked up every time it cries and falls back to sleep in a parent's arms, the association of being held while falling asleep is only reinforced, and it will be especially difficult to breakout of this habit. I am not suggesting that you ignore a baby's cries; it is vital to check that a child is safe and not hungry, sick, or needing a nappy change. The plan is to reassure the child, comfort them but not establish a model where they go to sleep in your arms. You can comfort a child with words, and/or by placing a hand on his/her back to show him/her that they are not abandoned, and then leave the room. This technique can take time, and you may have to return to the room many times, and it can be upsetting to hear a child cry and not automatically pick it up and cuddle it, but persistence will pay off in the end, and a better nights sleep for all concerned will be the reward.

Babies and children can suffer from disturbed sleep for many reasons, which will also disturb the parent's sleep in turn. Children's needs vary greatly from adults, but some babies and children naturally do not need much sleep, and they tend to grow into adults who also need little sleep.

Newborn babies can sleep 16 out of 24 hours, but they will wake periodically to feed or if they are uncomfortable or need a nappy change.

It is normal for a new baby to have erratic sleep patterns, but as the child settles down his or her sleep routine should become more regular. Many new babies are kept awake by colic; this may be because of wind, hunger or over feeding. During the daytime don't lay baby straight down to sleep after feeding, but keep them awake and amused for awhile until they sleep naturally, this may help prevent colic and the child will get used to being awake during the day and sleeping at night.

Whether a child sleeps alone, sleeps in the same room with other siblings or parents, or shares same bed with someone, it is important to establish a procedure that promotes sound, quality sleep. Older children with sleeping problems are usually children who haven't yet learned to sleep alone, or who have an anxiety problem. Fear of the dark, anxiety about school or separation from parents, or lack of a fixed routine before sleeping can all cause difficulties. A sleep diary kept by the parents for a few weeks should show up any pattern, and a simple remedy such as a night-light or an intercom can help. What is important is to recognize the problem in your child's sleep and to start to solve it. Intercoms are great for helping the child to feel in touch with the parents, and visa versa, but take care, it is easy to forget the intercom, and say something that the child or any other person shouldn't be hearing. Children do not benefit from being sent to bed as a punishment, it perpetrates the idea that the bedroom is hostile and not a place of rest. Ideally children should have their own room, or if they have to share, they should have their own part of the room in which they can put their own things, and create their own personal space.

There is a great deal of evidence on the importance of sleep for growth and normal development in children. Reports show that some abused children do not grow very well, probably because they are afraid to go to sleep or wake too frequently to have sufficient deep sleep, during which the growth hormone is released.

Children are very sensitive to arguments between their parents and major life crisis such as separation or divorce can make them feel anxious, restless and even feel responsible for the problem.

In all these situations love, support and reassurance is vital for the child.

Children's sleeping needs can vary just as much as adults do not try to force long sleeping periods on a child that does not need it. Many babies and small children naturally sleep for long periods each day, others do not. You must work around a timetable or routine based on your own and your child's needs. Formulate a simple bedtime routine, wash or bath, into pajamas, a story and then bed, and no late night adult TV.

Homework is best done early in the evening before or straight after the evening meal or teatime, and then there should be a period of play or relaxation before bedtime.

More care must be taken in using alternative remedies and therapies for babies and children. Never give a young child sleeping pills, alcohol or sedatives but try herbal remedies, and natural therapies like massage and reflexology. Babies and older children often love to be massaged or have their feet stroked, and they also like to reciprocate to others too. If they stay awake give them some stimulus like hanging mobiles, pretty pictures and colours over their cot or bed, and a teddy to cuddle. Many herbs are effective sedatives and will encourage wakeful infants to drift off to sleep. Valerian is particularly potent and has been used as a tranquilliser for over 2,000 years. It should be taken with the approval of a medical practitioner or herbalist. Infusion of passionflower, camomile or lime flowers can be very effective for children, sweeten with honey and give by teaspoon for babies and as sips from a small teacup for children over 3 years. Drops of lemon balm (Melissa) or passionflower tincture can also be added to warm milk or fruit juice. Hop, lime blossom and valerian baths have a very soporific effect.

Diet is also very important children could not have foods or drinks with high levels of caffeine or additives, coke, fortified orange drinks, before bedtime. A milky drink with a sweet biscuit has long been recognized as encouraging sleepiness. Milk is a rich source of the amino acid tryptophan, which the body converts into serotonin, a brain chemical involved with regulating the sleep patterns and feelings of tranquility. Other good sources of tryptophan are bananas, avocados, figs and pineapple. The mineral zinc may also be involved in healthy sleep patterns. Research shows that babies who wake one or more times a night between midnight and 7 am sleep more soundly when given 12 mg of zinc. Magnesium and calcium are often referred to as nature's tranquilizers. Calcium will also help with restless legs and growing bodies, (growing pains) which can torment older children and adolescents. A good vitamin and mineral supplement is advisable for all children with their sometimes fussy eating habits they may not be getting all the nutrients they need.

Homeopathy is very effective for children of all ages, and there are many remedies to treating sleeplessness, the following are recommended for children.

• Apis Mel, for the child that is tearful, fidgety and holds on to its urine in nursing infants. Shrill, sudden screams while sleeping or waking.

• Borax, for babies who wake shrieking from the slightest noise or for no apparent reason, or from a night terror. Or for a child that is asleep in your arms but wakes up when put in his/her cot or bed.

• Calc carb, for sleeplessness caused by stress or worry, with continuing unsettled thoughts and anxious dreams.

• Coffea, for children who sleep lightly, are very restless, waking at every sound, or unable to sleep because of excitement.

• Magnesia mur, for restless and anxious children, who toss and turn in bed and are very sensitive to noise, light or activity in the house.

• Stramonium, for babies who are terrified of the dark and wake up with nightmares, and can't be soothed by anyone.

• Sulphur, for the child that is difficult to calm, sulky or restless at night, kicking off the bedclothes, impossible to keep covered at night.

If buying over the counter remedies give 1 dose of the 30C remedy, wait to see if there is any improvement and, if so repeat to up to 3 doses. Or seek the help and advise of a qualified homeopathic therapist, always inform you doctor if you or your child is taking homeopathic medicines. (For more information on Homeopathic medicines see pagwes 223-226)

As a child gets older and needs less sleep, it is advisable to make sure that the child has something to do rather than packing them of to bed too early. Let them read until they are ready for sleep, I do not advise watching TV in bed as it is all too easy to fall asleep with in left on. If a child demands attention during the night, be firm with him/her that you must not be disturbed unless it is urgent, and supply the child with safe toys to play with until the child naturally goes back to sleep.

There is a difference, however, in the sound of a child crying simply to get attention, and the cry of a child who is genuinely afraid or unhappy. Children soon learn that their parents will be more sympathetic if there are physical symptoms such as headaches and stomach aches and will voluntarily of subconsciously manifest ailments to gain attention.

Problems where the child wants a parent to sleep in the same bed, can be taken on by sitting on the bed instead of lying down and, after a few days, move onto the floor beside the bed or a chair next to it, move until eventually physical contact will not be needed after the goodnight kiss.

Nighttime Eating/Drinking Disorder
This complaint signals excessive nighttime feeding with a baby or young child waking frequently during the night to be fed.

When children become hungry during the night they can wake up frequently, unable to fall asleep or return to sleep without being fed. A child who is used to being fed several times during the night may be accustomed to feeling hunger at those times without actually needing nourishment, and the parent's task will be to teach the child to feel hungry at more appropriate times of the day. It can be helpful to leave a drink and few grapes or a plain digestive biscuit by the side of the bed, and then the child can just help himself and not disturb his parents. A child who drinks and eats more during the night will also need to relieve themselves more during the night, resulting in more soiled nappies or bedwetting. Consult your doctor, midwife or baby clinic for safe and sensible ways to wean a baby or young child away from night feeds and into good sleeping habits and have him/her checked for illnesses like diabetes.

Sleep Walking

Many children and adolescents sleep walk, and it is very important that they are not woken suddenly or scolded for it when they do awake. It may be a sign of being unsettled, anxiety or worry about some particular incident. When the child is sleep walking just watch that the child does not hurt itself or wander into danger. If it is conceivable try to talk to the child the following day about what may be worrying or disturbing them, but try to do this without alarming or frightening the child. More boys than girls sleep walk, and it can run in families, as with adult's periods of sleep walking will be related to periods of anxiety or stress.

Nightmare and Night Terrors

Most children go through a phase of having nightmares and bad dreams and they usually go away naturally after awhile. Occasionally, young children may wake up in a terrified state, which then leads to continued sleep disturbance.

If the child remembers the nightmare the next day get him/her to talk about it and try to reassure him/her about any problems he/she may have or situations he/she finds scary of uncertain. Make the child feel as secure as possible and tell them they can always talk to you about their worries. The child going to bed feeling angry or distressed may cause night terrors. This can happen to adults too, and it is probably a reaction to some deeper worry that needs addressing. These night terrors can also be caused by low blood sugar, and will respond to having a high carbohydrate food such as a piece of bread or biscuit last thing at night. Don't give your child too much food or drink; however, as his/her digestive system will have to work overtime while he/she is trying to sleep. Using a safe burner or night light before going to bed with some essential oils can help with bad dreams, try a few drops of frankincense, cajuput or camomile for banishing old worries or apprehensions.

Teething

Children can be very fretful and even feverish when they are cutting teeth, but it does not always follow that these symptoms are due solely to teething. The first teeth erupt at an age when children are encountering infections to which they have not yet developed any immunity. The child may be teething or they may be ill, in either case it the child's sleep and yours will be disrupted and some measures need to be taken.

Homeopathic Chamomilla pilules can be a great help during teething. A couple of drops of camomile or lavender in oil rubbed on the child's cheeks or 4 or 5 drops in their bed time bath can also be very soothing and aid sleep.

Bed Wetting or Enuresis

Bed-wetting can be one of the banes of childhood; many children seem to go through periods of it at one time or another. It is more common in boys than girls, but tends to run in families. Most children gain control of their bladder as toddlers, three-quarters of children are dry overnight by the age of four years. However, the birth of a new baby can result in older siblings bed wetting, this can be an attention seeking ploy or a regression as a result of feeling put out or resentful of the new arrival. Pediatricians and psychologists have various remedies for it, some of which may work with some children and not with others.

It is a perplexing problem, embarrassing for the child and other siblings and aggravating for parents. Most experts agree that the problem is usually emotional or psychological rather than physical, although sometimes practical physical strategy's like having the child not drink water in the evening, having him/her urinate immediately before going to bed, or awakening the child up halfway through the night for a trip to the bathroom may prevent wet sheets in the morning. There are alarms you can buy that sound when the child wets the bed and these may help to re-train the bladder, also use incentives and rewards for dry nights. Never mock, deride or make fun of a child about their bed-wetting but stimulate progress with encouragement and rewards.

If an older child suddenly starts to wet the bed, when they have not previously had a problem, consult your doctor as there could be a urinary infection. Often the emotional causes rooted in stress and worry, these causes may have to be dealt with separately, or the anxiety will remain and can often lead to insomnia.

You may have to see a behaviour therapist to seek professional help, but many complementary therapies can also be of assistance.

Some children who wet the bed are prescribed imipramine (tofranil), a drug more commonly used to treat depression in adults. It has the side effect of improved bladder control, but should not be used for prolonged periods.

Reflexology before bedtime (regularly during the week) will relax and balance the child, helping them to cope with the deeper worries and tensions. There are also many other herbal and natural remedies that you can investigate, such as the herb Sweet Sumach taken as a tincture 10 to 15 drops three times a day.

If the problem is because of stress, tension or other underlying psychological problems you will be better off seeing a behavioural therapist, ask your GP for advise or referral.

Snoring and Sleep Apnoea in Children

Snoring in children should be taken very seriously, particularly if the child is sleepy during the day (or is hyper-active), aggressive, and has any learning difficulties.

Breathing movements might stop with mild obstructive sleep apnoea. In more severe cases the child's breathing can stop completely, to the extent that they wake up. Breathing often restarts with loud snores, mumbling noises, and grunting.

Food allergies should also be investigated as many young children have food intolerances that can affect their breathing by closing up the bronchial tubes while they sleep.

Natural Therapies for children

Natural, herbal and homeopathic remedies can often soothe an upset child and herbal drinks and baths before bedtime can be very beneficial. Massage, Aromatherapy and Reflexology are excellent ways of relaxing before bed. Children often respond well to Bach flower remedies and a drop of essential oil on the pillow can be very soothing. Take extra care when giving babies and children natural therapies, it is always advisable to consult your doctor, especially if the child has a medical condition or if they are taking any prescribed medication.

Aromatherapy and Children

Essential oils can have a positive effect on a child's emotional welfare. Babies and children are highly sensitive to smell, a few day old baby already associates mothers subtle skin scent with comfort, warmth, food and security. If you smear a few drops of an essential oil (such as rose or lavender) behind your ears, your baby will come to identify this aroma with you. Then if the baby finds it difficult to settle when you are not there, a few drops of your personal essence in the cot, on the pillow or teddy bear may soothe him/her to sleep. Some essential oils contain chemicals with are mildly sedative and can calm over excited children into restful sleep.

Smoothing a few drops of essential oils into the skin combines the benefits of massage and aromatherapy. As essential oils are very concentrated, they must always be blended with carrier oil before being used for massage. Never drop them directly onto the skin; the only oils that can be used directly on the skin are lavender and tea tree, for insect bites, spots or burns.

To dilute an essential oil add 1-3 drops of the essential oil to 5 ml of a carrier oil such as sweet almond, avocado, jojoba or grape seed. Essential oils are extracted from the flowers, leaves, stems and roots of aromatic plants; each essential oil has its own distinctive aroma and therapeutic properties. While many essential oils are used in perfumes and cosmetics we should never underestimate their therapeutic value. Many essential oils are good for stress, sleep, skin, repertory and digestive problems.

For newborn babies it is safest to stick to 1 drop only per 5 ml of camomile, lavender, or fennel.

With toddlers and younger children you can use 2-3 drops of camomile, lavender, fennel, sweet orange, eucalyptus, tea tree, peppermint or geranium. (See chapter 15 for more information on aromatherapy and some recipes for massage and bath, always use a lower dilution for a baby or a young child)

Suggested Visualization
Various relaxation techniques can be beneficial when sleeplessness is linked to stress and anxiety. Have the child imagine he/she is sleeping secure and safe at home, with his

parents sleeping contentedly nearby in their own room. If the child likes, he/she can also imagine the family home surrounded with a big, glowing white bubble that keeps them safe and keeps all the love inside and filters anything bad or troubling out and away.

Or if the child is good at visualization, let them simply imagine that their bed is surrounded by a big, glowing white parachute that keeps all harm away.

Children have brilliant imagination and they are often very good at doing visualization exercises.

When children have problems sleeping, they can be stressed, depressed or have low self-esteem, they lose trust in themselves, as well as in others, this can leave them feeling vulnerable and unprotected.

The following simple exercise can strengthen, protect and make one feel more secure, see if the child can do it on their own or they can do it together with a sibling or parent.

Find a quiet place, close your eyes, relax in a comfortable position, and let your breathing relax. Now imagine yourself standing before an open window, See a beautiful bubble come floating in, landing on the floor in front of you and growing until it is bigger than you, step into it, You are feeling totally protected, and you know that nothing and no one can harm you when you are inside your beautiful bubble.

Stress and Adolescents

Sleeping problems in younger children usually revolve around not being able to get off to sleep in the evening, but sleeping problems in adolescents may indicate something quite different. They may be getting enough sleep, but their sleep/wake cycle may often seem to be out of step with the rest of the world, they go to bed in the early hours and they don't rise before midday.

This can be infuriating, but isn't in itself a sign of anything more serious than that old generation gap or the adage of a rebellious teenager. On the other hand there can be emotional problems, tension and stress can affect many young people.

Stress respects neither social standing, sex nor age, and can affect young and old alike. Childhood days are supposed to be the happiest of our lives, but for many thousands of young people they turn out to be the most miserable, and the effects of a miserable childhood can last a lifetime. During childhood, the mental and emotional foundations of our lives are laid down; weak foundations leave a child emotionally and mentally vulnerable, often for the rest of their lives.

Some doctors estimate that one in ten children are suffering from depression. Stress can effect a child's psychological and physical development, it can manifest itself in bed-wetting, unruly behaviour, general lethargy, lack of communication and insomnia.

Distressed adolescents often grow up into distressed adults and their children are more likely to be disturbed. Having one depressed parent doubles a child's chance of developing depression before adulthood. Stress can leave children feeling isolated and unable to express themselves. Without help, either from parents or professionals, some emotional problems lead to serious disturbances and mental illness as adult. Common signals of stress in children are: aggression and bullying, eating problems, poor self-confidence, sleeping problems, social withdrawal and anti-social behaviour. Many of these problems can be difficult to treat, they can have physical symptoms like eczema, asthma, and stomach upsets, digestion problems and illness or many other psychological symptoms.

Get the advise of your medical practitioner or therapist, problems should be tackled early before they get out of hand.

Bullying

Bullying is a common cause of childhood stress and is much more serious than the usual playground teasing. While it can sometimes seem trivial to an adult, but prolonged bullying can destroy lives. The bullied themselves often become bullies in later life, when they themselves are put in positions of authority.

Bullying rapidly destroys a child's self-confidence, so address any bullying problem promptly, there is now much more awareness within schools and help is now more readily available.

Teenagers

Why do teenagers want to go to bed late and get up late, while many older people seem to feel ready for bed in the mid evening?

This could be because our circadian rhythms can get delayed when we are young, and advanced as we age.

Living with teenagers is often very stressful, but the same youngsters have their own problems. They have to deal with growing up, newfound sexuality, fresh responsibilities and independence.

They may also have to face the problems of drug use, peer pressure, racial harassment, bullying, a new job or unemployment. Parents have to come to terms with their children not being children any more but young adults.

114

Try to treat teenagers like responsible adults, talk to them calmly. Nothing winds teenagers up more than someone preaching at them all the time or treating them like an idiot. Make sure you answer their questions, especially about sex and changes in their bodies, honestly and openly. Remembers that teenagers may have completely different views from most adults about drugs, fashion and their environment. Try to build their confidence and self-esteem, being a teenager is difficult enough with out being criticized for the way you look and behave all the time.

Set rules but make them fair, be ready to make exceptions, be flexible, if you are too rigid they just won't obey anyway. Challenging rules is one way teenagers exert their independence. When things don't go to plan, don't overact, but try to talk things through and come to a compromise.

Remember your own teenage years and the problems you had, and remember that you are also a role model for your children.

Aim to be positive and approachable so that if they have a problem they know they can talk to you about it.

Teenagers often appear to sleep half their life away, but it is not uncommon for many young people to have sleep problems. Young girls worry about how they look, boy friends and all sorts of other things and teenage boys have very similar problems that they are not always ready to admit.

Negative self-image can lead to bulimia, anorexia nervosa, depression and suicide in the most extreme cases.

Bedtime Rituals or Routines
Sleep may be as natural as breathing, but good sleep habits have to be learned, parents can help by laying down good

sleep models for their child to follow in the future. A regular bedtime should be established as early as possible in the child's life.

Preparing a child for bed may mean separation of the child from his/her parents, and this can be a source of anxiety for many children and their parents. Parents naturally sense these disturbing feelings and want to comfort their children.

Make sure that the child is warm but not too hot, there are no draughts and that they have comforting toys to cuddle up to.

Many adults also find it a comfort to have an old teddy bear or something to cuddle up to in bed; we don't all have a partner to keep us warm at night.

If the child if afraid of the dark you can try a safe night-light to leave on in the room. If you check on the child during the night be sure not to disturb them by putting on a light or making a noise.

Bedtime should be a pleasurable and enjoyable experience for both parent and child, accompanied by story telling and plenty of cuddles. Bedtime can be one of the richest times for you and your children. When you plan your bedtime routine, it is important to set aside 15 to 30 minutes to do something special together with your child before bed. The activity should not be to stimulating (avoid bouncing, racing, or wrestling), nor should you tell scary stories or watch adult TV or videos. The child needs to know the time limits of this special time and that you will not exceed them. Giving in to requests for an extra drink or for another story, will teach a child that bedtime can be delayed. Without established sleep time routines, the evening is more likely to be filled with tension, anxiety and arguments.

Talk to your child even before he/she understands what you are saying, and listen to him/her when they can voice their worries and insecurities. Do not disregard any problems as silly or trivial, but address them together. Try not to scold or row with your child at bedtime and never send him/her to bed as a punishment. They may then associate their bed with correction, unhappiness and resentment.

If you have your own worries and problems, try not to show these anxieties in front of young children, at least not at bedtime. When they are old enough, talk to them and explain any difficult situation, the unknown is always far worse than the truth, if it is quietly explained.

If your child has severe sleep problems, regular nightmares, breathing or snoring problems consult your medical practitioner.

Some children who snore can have enlarged tonsils or adenoid problems. Make bedtime fun, most children love a leisurely bath time, with fun and games with mother or father. Add some lavender, juniper or camomile essential oil to the bath water (not more than 5 drops) to help the child relax. For most children a bedtime story is very enjoyable, they have one parent completely to himself or herself for a while, but be firm and don't give way when asked for just one more story, keep to a pre-arranged time scale.

It is important for parents to believe and understand the importance of limit setting during the day or night. For a child who won't stay in bed a reward system of positive reinforcement may also help. It is also important to discuss bedtime routine with babysitters, grandparents and other caregivers, so that the established routine remains in place consistently. When it is broken by prior arrangement for, holidays, special parties or visits to relatives, you must inform the child that this is a special exception.

Key Points for Good Sleep Routines for Children

- Keep to a consistent bedtime routine.
- Establish a relaxing setting at bedtime.
- Don't substitute television or video watching for personal interaction at bedtime.
- Avoid letting the child fall asleep with a bottle or while nursing, being held or rocked.
- Avoid food and drinks containing caffeine including colas and chocolate.
- Listen to your child if he/she has worries.
- Allow children there own personal space, even if they have to share a bed or a room with others.

According to a report by Dr Luci Wiggs, research fellow at Oxford University Children are sleeping for shorter periods of time each night. It seems that, 'go to bed' may no longer mean to go sleep, but rather, 'go to your bedroom and amuse yourself until you get so tired that you fall asleep with the video still running'.

One child in five is suffering sleep deprivation, which leads to symptoms that include short temper, poor concentration and low energy levels. Psychiatrists' say under 10s need between 10 and 12 hours sleep a night.

Her research shows that some children are getting as much as five hours less than their parents did at the same age. As I have said earlier in this book it is advisable to keep electronic equipment out of the bedroom if possible, space allowing have a separate room or separate area for TV and computers away from the sleeping area, this is doubly important for children. If this is not practical, then rules must be laid down and enforced, 'no TV after a certain time'.

Get back to that bedtime routine bath, milky drink, bedtime story, (for the tots), lights out and sleep.

Chapter 12

Relationships

Sleeping Alone or with a Partner

Sleeping with a partner can be advantageous, more people who sleep alone have sleep problems, but sharing a bed also has its liabilities. We have to adjust to sleeping with someone else, and sometimes our partner's habits can be disruptive.

We all wake up about six times a night even if we are sleeping well, although we will not always remember doing so. It doesn't take much of a disturbance to increase these numbers to a level at which the quality of sleep declines, and in many cases a partner may well be a primary contributing factor. If sleep schedules are a problem, try to agree on a mutually acceptable plan of action. If noise is the problem try earplugs, if one partner wants to read, get a light that shines directly down on one side of the bed, and try using eyeshades. Other possible solutions are to move times of intimacy to a better time, like early morning, or to ensure that the one who goes to bed later can get ready for bed without disturbing the sleeper. Snoring and sleep apnoea can be a problem and very disturbing, as discussed earlier, as can a partners restless limb movements in bed. If your partner tosses and turns at night and is also sleepy during the day, decide whether they may have a breathing problem at night or, indeed, a sleep disorder of their own. To minimize the effect of the disturbance, you could buy a larger bed, sleep in twin beds, or even sleep in separate rooms. Your objective must be to find a compromise, to be happy with your sleeping arrangements, having found an answer or solution to any sleeping issues that can satisfy both of you.

Relationship Problems

Most of us aspire to a loving, long-term relationship with one special person. As youngsters we dream of that perfect love, and then we grow up thinking of that ideal family. But the U.K. has one of the highest divorce rates in Western Europe, second only to Denmark, now four in ten marriages can expect to end in divorce. More than one third of all marriages involve at least one partner who has previously been divorced. All relationships and marriages go through bad patches, from minor tiffs to long-standing resentments that can make everyday life unbearable and restful sleep difficult to attain.

Do try to resolve your problems, or at least start to, during the day or early evening, don't leave it until bedtime to have rows. Children too can be very upset by parents rowing in the evening before bedtime. Every week nearly 3,000 children are involved in their parents divorce, with a third being under five. Children are very quick to pickup on emotional stress, it is better to tell them the truth, simply and straightforwardly, remembering not to blame either partner when there is a family breakup. Sometimes children feel they are caught in the middle of family arguments, and they can often hold themselves to blame in some way. Arguments in the home and stress between partners will often lead to restless nights for all concerned. When you have had a row or disagreement with your partner try to resolve it before going to bed, and don't lie in bed dwelling on your problems or fretting on what has happened between you.

Don't go into a relationship saying to yourself, I'll change him/her; you cannot change other people unless they want to be changed. People often have very false assumptions about what is going on in someone else's head. I don't want to start sounding like an agony aunt, but talk openly and honestly, share your feelings and worries, and listen to the other person's point of view. Nobody is perfect, we must all try to live together with our imperfections and learn to accept and love them as part of the person you adore.

Sex

It is generally agreed that sex, or making love with a willing partner is the one activity that is good to indulge in before bedtime. This would be on the assumption that you then drop off to sleep happy and relaxed. Sex should be relaxed, fun, satisfying and exhausting. Sexuality is a complex and sensitive thing, and lack of desire can have many different causes. It may simply reflect the sad fact that the one-time object of your desire has lost his/her charms, headache, and fatigue or there may be medical reason.

But an unsatisfactory sexual relationship can leave at least one partner feeling worse off than with no sex at all. As with all the other problems that cause insomnia, it is important to do something about it straight away, the longer any difficulty is left unresolved the more difficult it is to sort out. Insomnia and sleep problems can contribute to lack of sexual desire, if one is tired and irritable because they are not sleeping they are sometimes not going to want to/or have the energy to make love/have sex. The view among psychosexual counsellors is that most cases of low or reduced libido are due to:

• Harmful early influences, such as ideas received from one parent or other that sex is unpleasant.

• Anxieties, where one partner may be afraid of the other.

• Low stimulation levels, otherwise known as boredom.

Worrying about your performance in bed can cause stress and insomnia, as can the frustrations of the lack of or an unsatisfactory sex life. If you are alone you can still have sexual relief, yes I am talking about masturbation, there is nothing wrong with masturbating it is a safe and healthy release. Many people in relationships and out of them use sexual aids; these simple little devices help many women to reach orgasm. Sex toys are available by mail order and from some well-known commercial outlets. (Psychosexual counselling can untangle the psychological and physical causes of underlying sexual difficulties see useful addresses in appendix 1) Partnership problems are not always caused by sex difficulties, they can be brought on by many things. Stresses at work, a new job, unemployment, lack of communication, money problems, and difficulties with the children and many other things. You should strive to keep the romance in your relationship alive, make an effort every day, arrange special surprises for your partner, tell them you love them and don't ever take them for granted.

The following extract is from Susan Jeffers wonderful book *Opening Our Hearts to Men*:

How do we go about creating a love that really works?

It is about the story of the sculptor in India who was asked by an admirer how he was able to create such a magnificent shape of an elephant out of a piece of stone. The sculptor replies, "It was easy. I simply cut away everything that didn't look like an elephant!" Using this magical piece of wisdom as a model, I've learned that:

The way we create a loving relationship is to cut away everything in our actions and feelings that doesn't look like a loving relationship!

Abuse, Physical, Mental and Sexual

If you have suffered from or are suffering from abuse, be it physical, sexual or mental, do something about it now. Seek professional help, the victims of abuse often feel helpless and isolated, but there are many organizations that can help. Ignoring violence is dangerous, break the silence, living in a violent abusive relationship will destroy your confidence and make you feel that you have done something to cause the abuse.

The perpetrator of abuse may have often been the receivers of abuse themselves and may need counselling and help.

Violence in the home, or domestic violence may be slaps, kicks, rough handling, blows, shaking, rape, sexual in nature, even wounding or murder. It can also be mental cruelty, being humiliated or intimidated, being kept a prisoner in your own home or having food or medication denied. It happens in all social, cultural and ethnic groups and is usually directed against women or children by men, but not always. The abuser can be your partner, husband, wife, mother, brother, sister, son or carer.

In more serious situations a child or adult may have to be removed to safety and the perpetrator reported to the police or correct authority. Wife beating is now against the law; sexual abuse of any kind is taken very seriously these days, especially where children are involved. Even bullying at school or in the work place should be dealt with immediately and by the right authorities before it gets out of hand.

Look in your phone book for help numbers, go to the police, or local authority, citizens advise or your doctor, any of these will advise you where to get the right help for you.

If a child shows cruel destructive tendencies even from a very young age seek to find the reason for this behaviour and counsel the child. With the help of a behavioural therapist many problems can be nipped in the bud before they get too serious.

A child that kicks a flower one day, will hit a puppy the following day, and could harm a human the next. Respect for all nature and our fellow man must be instilled into our children from the very beginning of their lives, and remember that we all learn from the examples in our lives. Mental abuse can take many forms, from bullying, to just putting another person down all the time and telling them they are worthless. This can often be done subconsciously, constructive criticism is good, but continually telling some one they are hopeless and good for nothing is very negative and will lead to severe psychological problems in later life. Always try to find something good to say when you meet someone, no matter how bad things may be at the time there is always something positive to say.

Self Esteem

In cases where there is a dip in your self-esteem you must work at building up confidence and self worth. Get into the habit of looking after yourself and your family. Allow yourself a treat, wear your favourite outfit and don't wait for a special 'future' occasion to use those lovely lotions and potions that people have given you as gifts, treat yourself now and feel the better for it. If you find yourself bogged down with doing favours for other people all the time, running after a busy family and getting annoyed with yourself. Try saying no once in a while but don't shut yourself away from helping others and don't be afraid to ask for help, just give some time to helping yourself once in a while.

It's very important to let go of stress as quickly as possible, as it lowers your ability to take charge of your life, and consequently your self-esteem. Find a quiet, private spot, stretch your mouth as wide as you can and tense your facial, neck and head muscles. Then, clench your fists; beat the air and scream out load or silently depending on your surroundings. Start using positive language to describe yourself, avoid phrases such as, I can't do that, I'm useless, or I never seem to get anywhere. Try to replace them with positive affirmations such as I can do that, I will succeed, I am getting better, or I am happy and content. Turn problems into challenges and nervousness into excitement.

Not only will it help you, it will help your partner, friends and your children to lead a superior and more fulfilling life. If you feel good about yourself, and are positive about yourself you can be more supportive, understanding and giving to others.

Chapter 13

Women's Problems

It is undoubtedly true that women suffer more from insomnia and disturbed sleep than men do. This could be due to childcare, breast-feeding, menstruation, hormone imbalance, PMS and distribution of parental workload, but quite often sleeplessness is an indicator a longer-term problem. The National Sleep Foundation estimates that 40 per cent or more of women have trouble sleeping., compared to 30 percent of men.

Hormonal changes affect the quantity and quality of women's sleep. Women who suffer with PMS tend to get less REM sleep and deep sleep in the pre-menstrual period. As a result they do not get the quality of sleep they need and may feel extra tired and irritable at that time.

Research shows that 30-40 per cent of menstruating women suffer premenstrual tension and, indeed, some women experience very severe symptoms including chronic insomnia.

Hormones

Our hormones can have a big effect on the way we behave, so it could help us to understand how a women's natural cycle works. The ovaries produce two main female hormones, oestrogen and progesterone. Oestrogen controls the early part of the menstrual cycle, preparing the womb for the egg. Low levels can cause depression; high levels can cause short temper and irritability. Progesterone levels are high from mid cycle to end just before bleeding; it has a natural calming effect and is an important hormone if you are planning a baby. Some women who have PMS have been found to have low progesterone levels. During the lead up to the menopause, oestrogen levels can rise while progesterone decreases, leading to headaches, insomnia and mood swings.

Women also produce the main male sex hormone testosterone, which is responsible for energy and sex drive. Excessively low levels of this hormone can lead to a loss of libido.

Menopause

Menopause usually occurs around the age of fifty, but it can be ten years either way, like puberty it brings some dramatic changes to a women's body.

At menopause, the ovaries, which have been releasing eggs since puberty, shut down and stop producing the hormone oestrogen. Menopause does not happen overnight, for most women the process takes about five years with gradually diminishing menstrual periods. The symptoms can be disruptive and upsetting, menopause can affect some women's sleeping routine as hormones adjust themselves to pivotal changes in the body. Night sweats, hot flushes can be uncomfortable and annoying and the cause of sleep disturbance. Many women experience a short-term lack or sexual desire, depression, short-term memory loss and inability to concentrate.

Some of these symptoms are not due to oestrogen loss, but are simply a result of hot flushes and lack of adequate sleep. Some women find menopause a very distressing time, the realization that they have left their youthful years behind, they can no longer have children and the fact that their families have left home and may have families of their own and lives of their own. Menopause can also be a time of new beginnings, fresh starts, a time to try out new interests. It should certainly be a time to rejoice and enjoy new freedoms for women and not a reason to mourn and lament.

Menstruation
Menstruation is the periodic bleeding in women of child bearing age, when a girl is born her ovaries contain the bases of up to half a million eggs, which lie dormant until puberty.

From then until the menopause some 30 years or so later, an ovum is released each month from one or other ovary (ovulation), and finds its way to the adjacent Fallopian tube. The hormone progesterone, stimulates the lining of the uterus to form a thick layer, with an abundant circulation of blood, ready to receive and embryo it the ovum becomes fertilized, If no ovum is fertilized, the lining of the womb breaks away and is lost during a menstrual period. As soon as the bleeding is over the lining of the uterus regenerates, and some two weeks later the cycle begins again with the release of another ovum.

Premenstrual Tension, PMT or Premenstrual Syndrome, PMS
PMS, or premenstrual syndrome, was first reported in medical literature is 1931, and it has picked up a lot of attention in the past decade and has been viewed as everything from an illusion, to a defence for murder. PMS is in fact a hormone imbalance that manifests itself through a variety of symptoms. Hormonal changes affect the quantity and quality of women's sleep. Women who suffer with PMS tend to get less REM sleep and deep sleep in the pre-menstrual period. As a result they do not get the quality of sleep they need and may feel extra tired and irritable at that time.

Research shows that 30-40 per cent of menstruating women suffer premenstrual tension and, indeed, some women experience very severe symptoms including chronic insomnia. Many women who complain of PMS describe symptoms such as tension, mood swings, insomnia, irritability, anxiety, weight gain, bloating, breast tenderness, and cravings for different kinds of foods, (especially sweets). These signs manifest themselves a few days or one week before the period. Diet plays a crucial role in the treatment of PMS, and many women find increased symptoms of PMS when their blood sugar is not under control, hence the sugar cravings

Painful Periods (dismenorrhoea)

Some women have very painful periods; most women experience some pain, a slight dragging sensation, cramps and tender breasts.

Severe pain needing painkillers, and other symptoms such as fainting, vomiting or diarrhoea, could be considered to be abnormal and should be investigated by a doctor. Stress, other illnesses, insomnia, tiredness, poor general health and excessive use of stimulants all aggravate the pain. Conversely, relaxation techniques, tummy massage, physical exercise and sex and orgasms reduce it. I feel there is a strong built-in physiological element, that comes with the names we give menstruation, like the curse.

Missed Periods (amenorrhoea)

Primary amenorrhoea is when a woman has never had a period; secondary is when for one reason or another it has not come. Primary amenorrhoea is an abnormal condition and is very difficult to treat. Secondary amenorrhoea is generally due to some trauma, which temporarily shuts down the menstrual rhythm.

This can be caused by: weight loss, women under six stone do not menstruate because they do not have enough body fat to maintain a healthy pregnancy, which is why anorexic women often have no periods. Stress caused by a change of environment and the menopause is the other main reasons for missed periods.

Post-natal Depression

It is not uncommon for mothers to experience some depression immediately after the birth of a child. This can last days, weeks, months or in the worst cases even years if not treated. No doubt there are many psychological factors to consider, a new baby, a big responsibility, low self esteem (having lost your figure for a while), and the sleepless nights in the first months. However, many researchers believe that this post-natal depression is brought on by hormonal and chemical changes, which can be stopped with good nutrition and supplementation. One possibility is an excess of copper. The levels of copper tend to rise during pregnancy, while zinc levels tend to fall because the baby requires more. In most women the zinc content in breast milk declines rapidly as the infant uses up the mother's reserves. Depression is a classic symptom of zinc and B6 deficiency and new mothers should certainly take a supplement after giving birth. To help regain a slimmer figure, positive self-image and self-awareness new mothers can benefit greatly from massage, reflexology and aromatherapy. They must have some time for themselves even if it is only an hour a day to relax, pamper themselves and feel like their own woman again.

Osteoporosis

Osteoporosis is the thinning of the texture and weakening of bone, a condition so common in old people that it may seems an inevitable process of ageing. There is evidently some association with decreased production of sex hormones.

Women whose ovaries have had to be removed may develop osteoporosis at any age unless artificial hormones are given. An excess of adrenal hormones has the same effect. Anyone that is completely immobilized develops osteoporosis in time; the whole skeleton is weakened after a long period in bed. One factor is loss of calcium from bone, and it has been suggested that old people would be less liable to osteoporosis if they took more calcium in their food bones become brittle and break more easily. You don't often see men suffering from osteoporosis, though cases do occur. There are several reasons for this, men's bones are generally larger than women's and the amount of oestrogen circulating in their bloodstream is more or less constant throughout life. People who suffer from osteoporosis can have problems getting comfortable in bed and the constant need to move to get comfortable will also disturb sleep.

Exercise can help prevent osteoporosis especially weight bearing exercise. Our bodies were designed for plenty of physical activity, and some doctors believe that the rise in osteoporosis is due to our less active lifestyles. (see useful addresses in appendix .. for more information on osteoporosis)

Cystitis

Thousands of women and some men as well, suffer from cystitis. It is painful bladder infection, usually from bacterial infection, but sometimes from mechanical irritation from crystalline deposits in the urine. Cystitis is far more common in women than in men because infection frequently spreads upwards from the urethra (the tube that carries urine from the bladder to the outside of the body) and this is only about 1.5 inches long in women and four to five times that length in men, giving the bladder greater protection and because the anus is close to the urethra, which makes it easy for bacteria to reach the bladder. It makes people want to pass water frequently but, when they try, they can normally only pass a small amount of urine, and the act of urination causes a painful burning sensation. Cystitis can be brought on by sexual activity particularly if there has not been intercourse before or for some while, for this reason it is sometimes called 'the honeymoon disease'. It can also be caused by excessive consumption of a particular kind of alcohol or from catching a chill. Cystitis can seriously disrupt daily life and sleep patterns, frequent urination will disturb sleep and discomfort can keep you awake. Cystitis can be helped, and kept away, by drinking at least $1\frac{1}{2}$ litres of water every day.

Chapter 14

Sleep and Environment

Seasonable Effective Disorder, (SAD), Daylight, Sunlight and Fresh Air

There is a lot of interest in natural light and its connection to human health problems, like depression and insomnia. Biologists have discovered that not only is it vital for our well being, but that individuals requirements for light vary as much as individual needs for vitamins. As the human race become more 'civilized' they spend more time indoors. We travel to work by car, we work inside and we return home to sit and watch television. Children don't play outside but sit in front of televisions, computers or video games. There is no doubt that the shorter days of the autumn and winter months do affect some people adversely, they experience lethargy, lose of interest in sex, and develop depression. As daylight increases in the spring these feelings disappear and normal energy levels return. Whilst many people can say they feel a little down in the winter, there are some people who are so seriously affected by light reduction that they have a condition known as Seasonable Affective Disorder (SAD). These people become severely depressed, have joint pains, sleep problems, behavioural difficulties especially in young people, and digestive upsets. They may crave sweet foods and lack concentration to a conspicuous degree that seriously affects their work, and their lives.

They can also have difficulty sleeping and getting up in the morning and are often exhausted all day. Exposing the sufferer to ultra violet light or full spectrum light for at least 20-30 minutes per day can treat this condition. (see pages 208-209 for more information about light therapy and appendix 1 for stockist of UV light boxes) The light enters the eye and stimulates the pineal gland and inhibits the production of a substance called melatonin. Melatonin is normally produced at night in the dark and it makes us sleepy. Exposure to bright light in the morning boosts production of serotonin and encourages your body to use up more energy early in the day, so that you are ready to bed at night. Daylight is necessary for normal brain functioning and for the regulation of the sleep-wake cycle, so you can see that staying indoors when you are depressed or ill can make things worse.

If you work indoors all day try to go outside at lunch time, or at the end of the day, 20 minutes day light will have a greater effect that any pill. But you should also take a vitamin D supplement throughout the winter months to compensate for the lack of sunlight. Grapefruit essential oil used in massage, burners or bath is found to be very helpful for Seasonal Affective Disorder and depression.

Is your Bedroom Healthy?

In the last few years there have been many complaints of headaches, skin lethargy, depression, stress and insomnia that have been related to 'sick building syndrome'. The health of people in modern buildings has been affected by factors like artificial lighting, static electricity from synthetic fabrics, low frequency electromagnetic radiation and airborne particles. Air conditioning and non-openable windows further deplete the atmosphere of negative ions. Many of these factors can also affect your home and your bedroom. Don't use synthetic fabrics for furnishings, bed linen and nightclothes. Be sure to air your bedroom regularly and keep electronic equipment, TVs and computers, out of the bedroom if possible. Do without an electric blanket if you can, or at least make sure it is turned off before retiring.

Stress

Many people believe that viruses, bacteria and other foreign agents are responsible for many illnesses and ailments including insomnia, stress and depression. However, we are all constantly exposed to a wide assortment of hostile organisms, why are we not ill all the time? The idea of stress as a major factor in ill health is now becoming widely accepted. Stress can take many forms and will exacerbate any situation, making the individual even more prone to illness. Where there are inherited problems, for instance evidence shows that insomnia, asthma and eczema run in families, suffers know that any form of stress makes their symptoms worse. There are two parts to the body's reaction to stress: the alarm reaction and the resistance reaction. The alarm reaction is commonly referred to as the fight-or-flight response, because it initiated the bodily changes necessary to help us successfully run away or fight. The second part is the resistance reaction, which is slower and longer lasting. If stress continues for some time, the body remains in a state of apprehension and tension. This is when the body becomes vulnerable to sleeplessness, illness and infection. Although the effects of stress are becoming more familiar, what is not well known is the true range of causes, geopathic stress, for example, is usually ignored because most people are totally unaware of its presence. This type of stress is usually chronic, with exposure occurring every day, often for long hours as a person sleeps in a bed or sits in a chair above negative earth energies. The body is constantly fighting to cope with this on-going environmental stress by producing large quantities of the stress hormones.

Geopathic Stress and Ley Lines

The effects of geopathic stress can undermine and weaken a person's life force by weakening the body it then makes it more vulnerable to disease.

Geopathic stress consultants will set out to assess and deal with problems, which may be caused by the earths magnetic energy fields, and by electro-magnetic fields created by man-made objects like electricity pylons and wiring in the home. These energies can be generated by nature itself, from an underground river, nearness to geological faults in the earth's crust, or mines and old burial grounds.

In the home, televisions, computers, radios and other electrical appliances can cause geopathic stress fields to disturb your sleep, often because it give you headaches and make you restless and irritable.

According to geopathic stress consultants, geopathic energies pass through walls, windows, closed doors and other boundaries like fences and walls. Experts say there are many different types of geopathic stress, each affecting people differently, and possibly causing emotional or physical distress. They claim some people are more susceptible to geopathic stress than others. Geopathic comes from two Greek words: *geo*, meaning 'of the earth', and *pathos*, meaning 'suffering'. The word geopathic literally means suffering or disease of the earth, so geopathic stress is the general term for energies emanating from the earth that can cause discomfort and ill health in human beings. Another explanation for how geopathic stress affects the body is that the geopathic energies interfere with the bodies own electrical activity. The body itself contains many processes that are electrical, governing so much within our body, like the brain and heart beat. We are able to move our limbs because electrical messages are sent from the brain, via our nerves, to our muscles. Both sleeping and dreaming involve electrical activity within the brain, thus we are truly electrical creatures.

Ley lines are generally recognized as man-made phenomena, occurring where sacred stones, which have been charged energetically in some way, are laid in a straight line. You may hear people referring to all geopathic energies as ley lines, and this is misleading. A ley line appears 'naturally' and spontaneously if at least five such stones are placed in a line, with the two furthest stones no more than 25 miles apart.

Symptoms of sleeping over ley lines are; insomnia, restless sleep, depression on waking, exhaustion, and rheumatic aches and pains. There may obviously be other causes for these symptoms, I am not suggestion that geopathic stress is causing illness, but rather, it could be seen as a major contributing factor in many health problems including insomnia.

Consider the presence of geopathic stress if: you are not sleeping well, you are constantly restless, if you are not responding to treatment from homeopathy or acupuncture. If your cat regularly seeks out a specific spot to lie on, most plants and animals will not flourish in geopathically stressed areas, but for some curious reason they are favoured by ants, wasps, beetles, termites and cats. A responsive person feels a bad ambience in the room. A baby or a small child will sleep restlessly and or will move to one side or the bottom of his bed or cot in an attempt to escape the harmful radiation. An older child may wet the bed or suffer from nightmares.

You will need an expert with the correct machinery to detect ley lines and geopathic stress, and there are many devices now being sold offering protection against geopathic stress and or electromagnetic pollution. Many of them offer some protection against some forms of geopathic stress, but they can't protect against all forms of it.

PART THREE

Chapter 15

Remedies and Therapies to Aid Insomnia

As you've more than likely found out, it's rarely helpful to tackle your sleep problems in a halfhearted fashion. Remedies and treatments that ought to work don't, or they work for a while and then mysteriously, become ineffective. Your cupboards can become full of part used bottles of pills and your bank balance depleted from trying different therapies.

You will need to spend some money, but it is not necessary to rob a bank or take out a second mortgage to find out what is going to be effective for you. If you are going to improve your sleep you are going to need to be organized and methodical. Urgent problems must be dealt with quickly and the longer term issues tackled more comprehensively, this will take both time and planning.

There are two possible levels of action:

The first are the 'Contribution Factors,' past and present damage to sleep patterns, environmental components and health issues.

Here you will take immediate care of pressing problems. Here you must look at what is happening in your waking life, there may be issues you have to resolve, the things that happen when you're awake affect your sleep. If you are worried about a health problem, relationship or new job, then these things will need to be resolved or come to terms with.

Or you may feel healthy and can see no real problems that keep you awake, but your sleep patterns are out of synch. You will then need to look at your bedroom environment, bed position, and comfort and general ambience. Look at what you eat; drink and your lifestyle, keeping a sleep diary may be helpful here.

You may need to re-evaluate your actual sleep needs, don't assume that because other people you know need to sleep 8 hours, that you need to sleep 8 hours. You may only need 4 or 5 hours to function agreeably, and feel perfectly OK on only 4 or 5 hours. If this is the case make the most of that extra time, enjoy it and use it for yourself.

The second: 'Action, Rebalancing or Planning Stage', for better sleep, the emphasis here is adaptability, and performance, this might mean getting a few extra things done each week, or expressing your artistic or creative nature, even while you're coping with a busy life. Try some different approaches that you may not have considered before, open your mind to new ideas. What have you got to lose except bad old sleep habits, what have you got to gain except a new more fulfilling life and restful, refreshing and beautiful sleep. In part two of this book I have outlined many contributory causes and sleep disorders in part three I will give details of various natural remedies and therapies that can help you to build up a natural sleep cycle.

Try different things, keep a record of your successes and failures in a sleep diary, discover how to enjoy yourself and relax, learn from what you do and pass it on to others. You may find, for example, that giving a massage to a friend or loved one can be nearly as relaxing and pleasurable as receiving one. Learn to relax, take time for yourself and have your own space and time where you can be yourself. You will also find that with some homeopathic or herbal remedies you not only sleep better but you also feel more healthy and more able to face the world and its challenges. Meditation and relaxation techniques will calm your body and your mind and make you a more pleasant person to be with, you may find that your personal relationships will improve.

Exercise, even gentle disciplines such as Yoga or Tai Chi will make you fitter, you will feel healthier, your weight will be easier to control and you will have more energy.

Look at what you eat, when you eat, and what you put in your body, 'you are what you eat' this is true but you are also what you drink, smoke and anything else you abuse your body and mind with will have it's affects on your life.

The most important thing to remember is that it is not the length of your sleep but the quality of the time you spend asleep and how energized you feel in your waking life.

Relaxation Techniques

Relaxation techniques are just that, methods to help you relax. There are many different kinds, some help you relax your mind, others the body, although, I would say that the two are interconnected. A few relaxation disciplines see themselves as integrated systems for body, mind, and spirit harmony. Some focus on complete muscular relaxation, others promote concentration, while some also increase sensory awareness.

It is up to you to find the method that fits best to your needs, tastes and timetable.

Most of the following methods help you consciously relax muscles and balance your metabolism. Using words, breath, sound, or visual images, these structured methods help you focus on attending to body sensations, thoughts, or emotional states.

How Relaxation Techniques Work

Stress is the prime disrupter of our internal equilibrium, a disturbance in our natural homeostasis. The pressures of modern life and pollution in the environment can wear away at our bodies and our minds defences, leaving them unable to heal our bodies and so that they can then function wholly. Relaxation techniques help balance out the tensions and stresses so we are better able to cope; they calm us down, improve our rapport with our bodies, activate our self-healing mechanisms and reduce stress.

Doing relaxation techniques can only be time well spent, and often it is the taking a little time for yourself that is the most important object of the exercise.

Most relaxation exercises are easily learned, they are ideal self-help tools, and you can buy tapes and CDs, books, videos or go to classes. A stress reduction class may be a good place to begin learning the different kinds of relaxation exercises. Some kinds of stress can become chronic as sleeplessness takes a hold it can be a difficult process to reverse. Relaxation is not only meditation and deep breathing it can take the form of: hobbies, such as arts and crafts, reading, painting, exercise, walking, dancing, or any other activity in which you get away from your normal routine and relax.

Meditation

Meditation is undoubtedly one of the most effective ways to relax and build your defences against the daily onslaught of stress. Furthermore, meditation may help alleviate many stress-related diseases including hypertension, insomnia, and asthma. Classically, meditation involves sitting serenely, eyes closed, legs crossed, on a mat, but it can really be done anywhere, in a crowded room, at work or in bed. If you are doing meditation sitting up somewhere, you don't have to close your eyes, you can gaze vacantly or at a candle or a flower. Let your eyes be relaxed and unfixed, and preferably chose a time and place when you won't be disturbed. Meditation can be very effective once you learn how to do it, but you may need some guidance to begin with, look for a centre near you where you can find a teacher, most importantly you must feel relaxed, secure and comfortably with your teacher and confident in their ability to help you.

Relaxation Tapes at Bed Time

A large number of cassette tapes or CDs are available which can help you relax and reprogram your thoughts, some health food shops stock them, and meditation centres will have them for sale. You can buy various tapes or CDs on self-hypnosis, meditation and relaxation, and there are many books available on relaxation techniques. Many of these methods are a variation on the simple trick of counting sheep in various different visualization forms. I know that a lot of people do find meditation tapes at bedtime very helpful and there are many available, Some people favour listen to some melodious music or even a story tape or the radio, try out different things and see what is right for you.

In the 1960's many believed that you could learn while you slept, (Hypnopaedia), and courses for languages, self image, and many other subjects were available to learn on tape while you slept, I don't think that the results were spectacular or

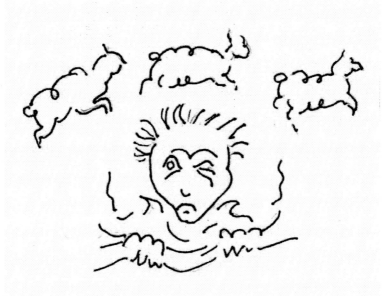

that any overnight geniuses or linguists have materialized from following this trend.

One thing I will say is make sure you have one of those tape decks that turn of at the end of the tape, and does not get stuck, or go click click click when they reach the end.

Leaving the radio on with the one-hour snooze switch turned on is also worth trying and has helped me in the past. Watching the television in bed is not a good idea, you will not sleep well with it on, and if you do go to sleep you will wake up to it flickering away and using up electricity. When you are listening to relaxation, meditation tapes or trying to concentrate on images of repose you will find that your muscles relax, you will begin to feel warm, drowsy and sleepy. You can do this in bed at night when you are ready to go to sleep, make sure that you are ready for bed and that every-thing is secure, so you don't have to get up again.

Creative Visualization

Complete relaxation is essential for conjuring up your imaginative skills and so is choosing the right image. The following images are only suggestions for visualization for inducing sleep or relaxation. If these images don't work for you, imagine any situation where there is cheerful noise and movement that gets less and less, for example:

• Imagine a tree filled with songbirds. The birds fly away from the top branches, then the next branches, and so on until there is just one bird left. Concentrates on him until he flies off, then look at the branch he was sitting on, and then let your mind focus on just one lovely pale green leaf.

• Or think of a playground of noisy, tumbling children. It's suppertime they gradually go home. Watch the last child as he goes off with his mother to have his tea and then go to bed, he looks very sleepy.

• One technique that helps many people is to imagine lying on a warm beach, see the palm trees blowing in the breeze, hear the waves gently lapping at the shore. Breathe deeply letting your breaths go in and out slowly in time to the rhythm of the waves. Think of your toes and feel them warm and relaxed, follow this pattern throughout your body. Up through your legs, your fingers and arms, then into your lower body and abdomen. Slowly feel the warmth of the sun lull you and your breathing becoming deep and slow. As you come up through your lungs, shoulders and head allow yourself to slowly drift away, casting aside all your cares and worries.

If you have trouble quieting your mind with images, try concentrating on the feeling in your nostrils as your breath enters and leaves your lungs. Or still the mind by repeatedly saying or thinking a simple word or sound, or counting to ten, or back from ten to one over and over again. One old wives tale I heard that does often work is to think of black, just visualize a black canvas, in this way you can block out any other obtrusive thoughts that may disrupt your mind and stop you from sleeping.

Passive Hearing and Active Listening

This is a relaxation technique that you can practice anywhere, at a party, a room full of people, waiting for a bus, alone at home or when trying to sleep. Get comfortable with your neck, head and chest in a straight line and keep your mouth closed.

Close your eyes and concentrate on all the sounds you can hear around you outside the room, try to shut out all other sounds. Try to identify the sounds you hear and decide what is the cause of them. When you are fully aware of sounds outside, switch your attention to the sounds in the room and those closer to you. After awhile turn your attention to the sound of your own body, your breathing and the sound of your heart beat, feel yourself merging with those sounds.

If you are really listening actively you should be aware of how loud you're breathing and heart beat sound now compared to how they were at the start of the exercise. This exercise demonstrates the difference between passive hearing and active listening, and can help you relax and tune into yourself.

Deep Breathing

One of the main reasons many of us are tense is our shallow breathing, most people breathe very shallowly, using only the top part of their lungs. By breathing deeply and providing more oxygen to our bodies, we are energizing and rejuvenation every organ and cell in our bodies. It is one of the most effective and beneficial methods of relaxation.

Lie on your back comfortably, and slowly relax your body, starting with your feet and moving through every part of your body until you have reached and relaxed your face and scalp. Then, slowly, begin to inhale, first filling your lower belly, then your stomach area, and then your chest and the top of your lungs almost up to your shoulders. Hold for a second or two, then beginning to exhale, gradually building up the time between breaths to 5 or 10 seconds. Empty the very bottom of your lungs first, then the middle, then finally the top. Continue this breathing for 5 to 6 minutes making the in and out breaths longer as you progress, the out breaths should ideally be slightly longer than the in breaths. After a while, imagine that you are resting on a warm, gently ocean. The sun in shining peacefully on your body as you rise and fall on the gentle swells of the water, you rise up on your inhale, and slowly descend on your exhale. As you do this, concentrate on a spot on your lower belly near your navel, you may find it helpful to put a hand on your stomach and feel the rise and fall as you breath. The stomach is the centre of gravity in the human body, as discovered and used over thousands of years by oriental martial arts disciplines and used in yoga and meditation techniques. Feel the energy from that point gently flow out and fill your entire body with peace and serenity.

Continue this relaxing breathing and combine it with any of your visualization techniques, use with one of your affirmations, or if you want to until your fall asleep. Full breath breathing aids digestion and sound sleep. Use it when you need to calm down or think clearly. Use it when you feel depressed or unhappy. The next time you see a baby or a small child asleep, notice the way she/he breathes. How is this different to the way in which you breathe? The full breath is also known as 'soft-belly breathing' because it promotes the relaxation of the abdomen and prevents the tense, hard-belly approach to body posture. Posture echoes our mood and attitude. And it can also affect both in a positive or negative way. The Soft-belly posture allows you to remain calm and balanced, to breath more deeply and maintain a centre of gravity below the navel.

146

Meditation and Yoga are relaxation techniques that have been with us since ancient days. Christian, Jewish, and Eastern religious traditions all include some type of meditation, usually associated with their respective mystical traditions, often though of as prayer. Many forms of relaxation contain an element of exercise as part of the relaxation process.

Exercise

People who do physical work outdoors like farmers, fishermen, and construction workers often find they get enough fresh air and exercise, and can be more sleepy at the end of the day. It is proven that people who get more exercise during the day enjoy better sleep at night, because sleep is the natural response to physical tiredness. Physical activity can be anything from walking to gardening, climbing a flight of stairs instead of taking the lift and taking part in sports and exercise classes.

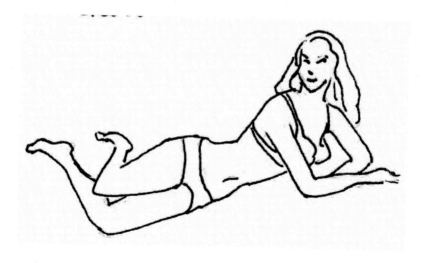

Exercise will energize you, it will help you lose weight, it will help with the diseases of ageing, i.e. osteoporosis and arthritis, and will decrease your stress levels and help you sleep. It is probable that the rise in temperature produced by exercise, promotes sleep, increasing the metabolic rate and improving the internal rhythms of the body.

Don't engage in any new or strenuous physical exercise if you have doubts about your health, for most people it is wise to have a medical check up before starting a new exercise programme. The best time to exercise is in the morning, late afternoon or early evening and if you can combine getting some exercise with some fresh air so much the better. Some gentle exercise, like yoga, one hour before bedtime can help some insomnia sufferers. Vigorous exercise delays the secretion of melatonin, the hormone that is responsible for preparing your body for sleep, so exercising within four hours of bedtime will hinder you from sleeping. Join a gym, yoga class, go swimming or go for a brisk walk, if it is possible rope in a partner or a friend, it is always easier to keep the momentum going with a mate or partner to spur you on. Don't try to do too much too soon but gradually build some regular exercise into your life. A walk in the fresh air every day will do you a lot of good, and clear your mind as well as exercise your body. Sex is also a good form of exercise and one that can be practised at any time of the day or last thing at night before sleep.

Even the elderly, physically weak and wheelchair bound should get some exercise, Ta'i Chi is good or try my 10-point flexibility plan in appendix 3.

There are also gentle exercises that the bed ridden or physically disadvantaged can do with the help of a friend, family member or carer.

Fresh air is vital to good health and a clear mind; take a walk, no matter how short, in the fresh air every day if you can. A friend of mine lost two stone and said she had never slept so well in her life after acquiring a dog and taking him, or him taking her, for a walk each evening.

T'aí Chí, Aíkíðo, anð Other Martíal Arts

Martial arts are systems of physical and mental training used for self-understanding, expression through movement, and self-defence. Primarily Asian practices, they are also found in other parts of the world such as South America and Africa.

Martial art developed out of ritual dances and diverse forms of combat, hand-to-hand, work, spear or staff. The most popular philosophies and martial arts techniques developed in China and Japan.

Some martial arts available in the West today are:

Aikido (Japanese), Chi Gung or Qi Gong (Chinese), Judo (Japanese), Jujitsu (Japanese), Karate (Japanese), Kendo (Japanese), King Fu (Chinese), Tae Kwon Do (Korean), T'ai Chi Ch'uan (Chinese), Kalinda 'stick fighting' (Africa and the West Indies).

Some advanced forms of martial arts train their students in healing techniques, channeling the life energy forces of chi, and ki. The roots of many martial arts reach back to ancient ritual dances from more than 5,000 years ago. Dances would celebrate folk heroes and nature, as well as animals and had many gestures that became the bases for some yoga exercises. These movements can balance organs, relieve leg cramps, uplift the mind, and relax the body. In China you will still see the early morning streets lined with old and young alike doing their T'ai Chi exercise movements as a start to the day.

Training in the martial arts can be healthy for the mind, body and spirit. Chose one that fits your personality, health needs and values or philosophical orientation. Karate, Judo, and other competition-based forms are vigorous self-defence and strengthening exercises.

T'ai Chi and Aikido

T'ai Chi, is the most gentle and personal of the arts, it is a form of meditation while in motion and very good for calming the mind and body. Chinese doctors often prescribe T'ai Chi as complementary treatment for stress, nervous conditions and insomnia; it is suited as a health practice for the weak, elderly, and infirm. It improves blood and lymph circulation, and the increased energy flow also helps ward off illness and fatigue. Like T'ai Chi, Aikido stresses "non-doing" letting the body act in a smooth and natural way that reduces habitual tension. Both use fluid and circular movements and emphasize personal development and awareness and treat the mind and body as one.

There are numerous Keep Fit, Yoga, T'ai Chi, and other martial arts classes around and many schools, colleges and evening classes will do introductory sessions so you can get a taster before committing yourself to a prolonged period of classes, go and explore find what is right for you. The benefits of practising a martial art can reach beyond physical well being they can help with mental alertness, and relieving stress in your life.

Yoga

Yoga is one of India's wonderful gifts to mankind. Yoga's most valuable quality is that it builds up a store of physical health through the practice of a system of exercises called asana, which, keep the body cleansed and fit. Yoga believes that exercise is essential for speedy removal of toxins and for keeping blood circulation and all internal processes functioning smoothly. Yoga really helps the mental state, there are different breathing exercises or techniques to calm the mind and brain, offering inner peace and an ability to face upheaval and deal with problems that can cause insomnia. There are many different types of yoga but the most appropriate for insomnia is Hatha yoga, which incorporates relaxed health, harmony meditation and relaxation.

Your Special Place

Everybody must have their special place, we have all at one time in our lives had a special place, where we felt calm, safe and at peace. Try to remember this safe haven when you want to feel secure, use it as your refuge at times of stress or when you want a few minutes peace and quiet. If you can't think of a real place and time make one up, it could be a special secret garden or a quiet glade in the woods filled with blue bells. Just use your imagination and come up with something special to you and to you alone. Use this special place when you meditate, do your relaxation exercises or just when you want to feel calm for a minute. Lie down with your eyes closed and imagine you're in your very favourite, most peaceful place, It may be a sunny beach, swinging in a hammock in the woods, by a river, your own back garden, or on top of a mountain. Where ever it is, imagine you are there, you can see and feel your surroundings, hear the peaceful sounds, smell the fragrance of the flowers, and feel the warmth of the sun or whatever other sensations you are imagining, relax and enjoy.

In addition to your very own imaginary special place your must have your own safe corner in the real world, it can be difficult in this busy world with limited space, a busy life or noisy family to find your own special place. Try to find an area that is yours; fill it with things that are special to you, photos, favourite mementoes, crystals or a flower in a vase. Make the family aware that this is your special place and that they

151

must respect it and your time when you need to be left undisturbed.

Choose a specific time to be alone with your thoughts every day and make it known that this is your time, and you are not to be disturbed, unless the house is burning down.

Paradoxical Intention

This is a technique developed to help you sleep. It works by using a contrary suggestion. You concentrate on remaining awake and are resolute that you will not go to sleep. It helps some people, presumably by blocking out disruptive thoughts that are keeping you awake. Or you can visualize someplace that you have always found extremely boring, a teacher or relative who was so boring that he/she almost puts you to sleep, a long train journey with the same scenery going past the window, or a wearying task you have to perform. You can also imagine that it is time to get up, the alarm has gone off and you're not allowed to sleep any more. You know how delicious that feeling is in the morning when it's time to get up but you're still so tired and your eyes are heavy and you shouldn't do it but you just want to snuggle back down in the covers and sleep for a few more minutes.

Quiet Ears

This technique comes from an Ancient Eastern meditation, you must lie on your back with your hands behind your head, fingers interlocked, and your palms cupping the back of your head. Place your thumbs in your ears so that you are pressing the outer flap of your ear and blocking the entrance to the ear canal. Then lie quietly and listen for a high-pitched sound that you will gradually hear inside your head. Concentrate on the sound as in the active hearing and passive listening exercise on page 145.

Just lie there for 10 minutes and concentrate on that sound and only that sound, then lower your arms and breath deeply and calmly, relaxing your mind and body into sleep. Take care with this exercise if you suffer from tinitus, although it can help some people to control the noises that they hear involuntarily and that can cause such distress.

Affirmations

One of the best ways to break unhelpful sleeping habits is to begin exchanging them for helpful ones. The very first thing is to recognize in what particular ways your accustomed thinking or behaviour is keeping you in that sleepless mode. How do you talk to yourself and others about your sleep, do you say 'I am an insomniac', do you expect not to get a good nights sleep, and tell other people this. If you do, you are reinforcing this expectation onto yourself. You don't expect to sleep well; therefore, you won't sleep well. You can change some of your thinking now, by telling yourself that you are now on the way to improving your sleep, and by no longer telling other people that you suffer from insomnia. Many people enjoy having something to complain about, and their ailments give them something to talk about. In many cases this can be an excuse for avoiding other issues, things not right in their lives, of a sign of the boredom or lack of interest in their life. If this is true of you, do something about it, and do it now. Join an evening class, join a gym, take up a hobby, spend more time with friends or family, read, or write a book.

If you have family commitments get them involved, or if they don't want to be involved demand some time just for yourself. Start noticing your habitual thoughts about insomnia, look out for sentences like: 'I always take ages to go to sleep' or 'I always wake up at 3 am and can't get back to sleep'.

These statement may not be true, it may feel true to you, but the fact is you don't always wake up a 3 am and do not always take ages to go to sleep. You have to start making positive affirmations.

Here are some examples:

• I am going to sleep peacefully throughout the night and I will wake up at 7 am refreshed and ready to face the day.

• I will sleep, dream of beautiful things and be restored in the morning.

• My sleep will be restful and peaceful; I am in control of my life, body and mind.

By starting to change your attitudes, the way you talk about yourself and see yourself, can be an astonishing way of opening up other possibilities in your life. Once you realize that you don't have to be a victim of your own thinking and reactions, all kinds of barriers can begin to crumble.

Your might try writing down one of these affirmations, or making up one of your own, and putting it under your pillow when you go to bed, add a drop of lavender or camomile essential oil for good measure, and go to bed with a positive mind.

Take each night as it comes and don't expect things to change overnight, they will change, but you may have a lifetimes conditioning to overcome so be patient.

Pain Resistance Exercise
If pain is one of the reasons for your insomnia try the following colour relaxation technique for pain relief. There are two possible ways of dealing with pain: to accept it and relax in to it, or to focus your mind on something completely different. Although these two methods might seem

contradictory, what they have in common is that both remove the resistance to pain. Resisting pain always makes it worse; tensing up against it tightens muscles and restricts the flow of blood. Mentally resistance also makes it worse. Alternatives are to learn how to relax into the pain, accepting it as a bodily sensation, breathing into the pain and letting go of the pain as you breath out. Use imagery while you relax, perhaps visualizing the pain as a blob of colour, which slowly dissolves, going out of the body through your fingers and toes. Focus on something other than the pain, so long as it's something pleasant, imagine yourself in beautiful surroundings, or remember a place where you have felt happy and peaceful, your special place.

The Legend of the Dream Catcher

Dream catchers are a Native American tradition based on the belief that dreams are filled with meaning and intent. Native Americans designed and make use of dream catchers so that no fundamental message contained in their dream would be lost.

Legend has it that day and night the spider woman wove tiny dream catchers on the tops of cradelboards to make certain that babies slept peacefully. Bad dreams became entangled in the web and only the happy ones filtered through. The sleeping babies laughed and clapped their hands for joy and no harm ever came to them. With the first rays of the sun, the bad dreams broke free and returned to the place of shadows.

The design of the dream catcher is a hoop with crystals, feathers and beads attached, joined to a web net with a hole in the centre. It protects you from harm while you sleep, catching the good dreams as they pass by and getting rid of any bad dreams as they drop through the holes in the middle. Hang your dream catcher from the ceiling above your bed, allowing your dreams to pass through it.

The dream catcher is said to be a great antidote against insomnia and restless nights. Personalize your dream catcher by putting something of your own on to it, a piece of jewellery such as an odd earring, a snip of your own hair or piece of ribbon.

You will sleep easier and have wonderful dreams that may hold some wonderful significance in their message.

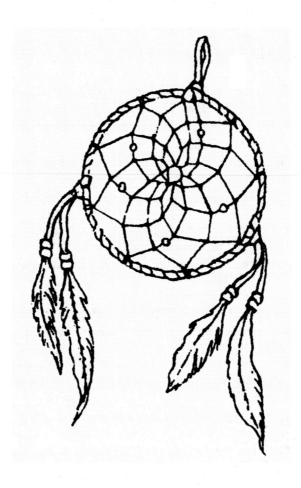

Chapter 16

Mind Therapies and Healing

Hypnosis or Hypnotherapy

History

Hypnosis is a phenomenon that is within the everyday experience of everyone. It is seen as a novelty act in shows, and is often seen as connected to the occult and more sinister mind control. In clinical hypnosis, the therapist enables the client to enter into such an altered state of awareness for the numerous therapeutic benefits that it makes accessible. The ancient Greeks use a phenomenon like hypnosis to cure anxiety and hysteria. In the late eighteenth century, a Viennese physician, Franz Mesmer, successfully treated many people by putting them into a deep trance. The real founder of modern hypnotherapy was Dr Leibault, he wrote the fist major book on hypnotism, and maintained that it could help many medical conditions. Hypnotism came to the UK in the late nineteenth century by James Braid, a Manchester surgeon but was not approved by the British Medical Association until 1955. Since the 1970s hypnosis has been more recognized and is now used in practice by the NHS in the UK and many other parts of the world.

Theory
Hypnosis is not sleep; neither does the therapist take control of your mind. At all times the client remains in control, whilst the therapist acts as an intermediary. You cannot be made to do anything, whilst in the trance state, which is against your will or your moral, religious or philosophical standpoint. Increasingly people in the West are beginning to trust in the power of the subconscious and use it to improve mental and physical health, and to gain control over their lives.

Hypnosis, which taps the power of the subconscious and uses it to shut out pain, fight disease, and even stimulate cell renewal, is one way in which many people have learnt to use the power of the mind to heal themselves.

It is used to help clients to stop smoking, stop nail biting, assist with weight control, treatment for addiction to drugs and alcohol, and to reduce stress and anxiety levels. If an underlying problem is stopping you sleeping, from worry or physical symptoms hypnosis can be a useful tool in unlocking that problem. Hypnosis can often be used for regression, and can unearth problems and traumas that you may have a hard time, or hard work dealing with.

Treatment
After an initial consultation on general health and psychological state the client will be induced into a relaxed state of mind, they may be fully aware of what is going on or they may feel as it they have been to sleep for a little while.

Relevance to insomnia
Hypnotherapy can without doubt remove blockages that may cause insomnia; it can uncover hidden worries and stresses and relax the mind. It can also plant suggestions of restful sleep in the mind so that it is easier to obtain.

Warning
Think carefully before embarking on this road, you may uncover some stuff that you hadn't bargained for, and you must always check that you are seeing a qualified and registered therapist.

Eye Movement Desensitization and Reprocessing, EMDR

History
EMDR was discovered and developed by Dr Francine Shapiro. In the USA, who describes walking in a California part in 1987 and being troubled by disturbing thoughts. She noticed that her eyes were spontaneously moving horizontally back and forth in what are called saccadic eye movements, and that after this had occurred she felt better. She began to incorporate eye movements into some of her therapeutic techniques with good results, and the used the eye movements systematically in some formal research for post traumatic stress disorder. The results of that study were published in 1989 and it was established that EMDR could help people suffering from trauma, stress and painful memories. EMDR treatment has grown rapidly since 1989 and well over 600 British clinicians have now been officially trained in the therapy.

Theory
REM, the period of deep dream sleep helps the mind work through distressing memories. If this REM process doesn't occur after a traumatic episode, the mind can hold on to the emotion. Leading to problems. This is where EMDR helps but you do while you are awake.

The dual focus of thinking about the negative memory and following the therapist's finger can literally push the locked information along the brain's information processing system to accelerate the healing process.

Treatment

The therapist will take a thorough case history and discuss the initial traumatic experience and resulting symptoms. You will then be asked to focus on your anxiety or problem and bring to mind an image that may have represented the fear or problem. The therapist will then give you a positive thought to hold on to in your mind, such as I will sleep peacefully without a nightmare' as you watch the therapist's finger move from side to side and lift to right. The mind doesn't go into a hypnotic state but it does increase brain activity.

Relevance to insomnia

This therapy can help with disturbing memories and nightmares after a traumatic experience and some phobias like claustrophobia, bereavement, stress and low self-esteem. It is widely accepted that symptoms such as "flashbacks", avoidance behaviours cause sleep difficulties and are emotional numbing following trauma. EMDR can certainly help with insomnia in these circumstances.

Warning

Not suitable for those suffering from epilepsy, poor ego, psychotic problems or severe depression, and taking depression medication. Severe Obsessive-compulsive disorder can be difficult to treat as can many mental disorders.

Psychosynthesis Counselling and Psychotherapy

History

These are all therapies that come out of human analysis, via Freud. Sigmund Freud changed medical and mental health history by inventing psychoanalysis, the long-term, verbal treatment of physical, psychological, and emotional problems. Counselling (in psychology), guidance offered in the form of discussion rather than any specific type of therapy. Counsellors may have a quantity of specialized knowledge on particular problems, possible solutions, and the potential pitfalls of different solutions, but often they see their role as assisting those who consult them to find their own solutions. Counselling may be available to help people adapt after physical injury, traumatic shock, when a family has been incapacitated by mental or physical injury, when a marriage is unhappy, or when a child has been abused. It may be offered by psychologists, doctors, social workers, or trained lay people. Counselling should be distinguished from psychotherapy, although there is some overlap. It is less intensive and sometimes more directive, and its clients may have a much wider range of concerns for which they require guidance.

Theory

Traditionally psychotherapy has attempted to trace the origin of disease in order to take remedial action. Psychosynthesis agrees that whilst the source of many symptoms may be located in the past, not all distress can be explained in this way.

Some symptoms such as lack of meaning in life, alienation, or loss of identity, may not be of a neurotic nature but point rather to existential crisis. The symptoms therefore carry within them positive messages that are seeking to express themselves in our lives. It is the appreciation that a symptom contains meaning and can be a healthy phenomenon that the psychosynthesis approach has to offer. Therapist would work one to one in a counselling situation and can help their client to come to terms with their problems.

Treatment
The therapist will take a comprehensive consultation of health and mental data, and will then by using leading questions attempt to get the patient to talk, and to relax, and to uncover any past problems or traumas that may be affecting their current health and state of mind.

Relevance to insomnia
These therapies can be very helpful to insomnia sufferers, but it will depend greatly on what is causing the insomnia or sleep problem. It nightmares, depression or nervous tension is being caused by underlying worries or psychological problems then councelling or psychotherapy can help release the tensions that are causing the sleep problems.

Warnings
Treatments can bring up stuff that has been long buried and that will have to be dealt with, this can be a very expensive therapy as the patient may need treatment in the long term, some times for years.

Bioenergetics and Body-Oriented Psychotherapies

History
Psychotherapy, the treatment of emotional or behavioural problems by psychological means, often in on-to-one interviews or small groups. Freud devised the first systematic

approach, initially discussing patient' problems with them, but later allowing theme to do most of the talking in a procedure called free association of ideas. This has been the model for subsequent psychotherapies. These therapies were developed at the turn of the century when there was a new awareness of self and society had shifted away from puritanical and Victorian repression.

One area in which this new freedom was manifested was a growing interest in the radical science of psychiatry. One pioneer, Dr George Groddeck, proposed that sources of mental illness lay deeper than the conscious mind. In a pre-Freudian view of the unconscious, and he incorporated body manipulation and other activities into his therapies. Reichian theory, based on the original thinking of radical psychoanalyst Wilhelm Reich, explores the heeling capabilities of the body. Bioenergetics is an offshoot of the original Reichian therapy. Combining eastern philosophy with western body oriented psychotherapy theories.

Theory
Body-oriented psychotherapy is an offshoot of traditional psychotherapy, a primary treatment for mental illness that helps individuals cope with and resolve psychological and emotional problems. It can be a more invasive therapy involving dance/movement, and physical contact, the therapist applying strong pressure on the patient's chest, or nurturing or gently holding the client releasing the inner tensions and memories that are causing problems.

Off shoots of this therapy are "talk therapy" and "dance/movement therapy" these therapies are frequently practiced separately. (also see Rosen Method page 178-180)

Treatment
After an initial consultation of general health the therapy involves, deep breathing, massage, vocal exercises, stamping, kicking, and other stress releasing techniques. It is vital that the therapist can create a rapport, trust, and strength in a relationship. In Bioenergetics the patient uses mat on the floor, a chair, a stool and blanket, or simply stands free. Sessions can alternate between using stress position exercise to open up muscular emotional blocks, and talking about what is causing those blocks.

Relevance to insomnia
This therapy is very effective where there are underlying traumas, doubts, and painful memories that may be contributing to sleeplessness.

Warning
The effects of body-oriented techniques can be unexpected and powerful, always make sure you work with a qualified therapist, who you can trust completely. Patients can manifest physical symptoms and side effects such as; migraines and headaches and allergies.

Healing

History
There are many kinds of healers: people trained in esoteric knowledge, those possessed by the spirit of a dead person, individuals adept at channeling a special quality of energy, and/or persons drawing on the power of a faith.

The Western traditions of healing are wide-ranging and have many labels: Absent healing, clairvoyant diagnosis, energy healing, faith healing, magnetic healing, laying-on of hands, psychic healing, psychic surgery, and spiritual healing.

Healing is one of the oldest professions in the world; every village East and West would have the local healer, who could be a priest/priestess or local wise person. Often this local village person would have knowledge of herbs and other arts, and sometime they would be called a witch and persecuted by the community.

Theory
Healers in each of the categories draw on the help of powers of beings from another realm or reality. Whether invoking the grace of God or religion, or clairvoyant knowledge, these men and women gain their power in some unplanned way, by years of spiritual training or they are born with it. But the fact is they would often be consulted with successful results, when all else had failed, and their potency is in the power of belief. Healing can be very effective for complains such as AIDS, cancer, diabetes, and sources of all illnesses that are associated with a spiritual problem.

Treatment
Treatment will involve laying hands either on or just above the body in different positions or just above the persons head, this enables the healer to give the patient energy through themselves to help to cure or restore the body or mind of the patient.

Relevance to insomnia
As healing in theory can help any disorder of mind or body it can then help with insomnia, it will certainly do no harm.

Other information

There are many different kinds of healing:

• Spiritual healing and Spiritualist healing: These healers see themselves as the conductors of supernatural healing forces, or energy some go into a kind of trance. They channel this energy into the patient by laying their hands on or around them in order to rebalance the body and promote healing.

• Aura healing: Auric healers are able to see an aura, or ring of colour, that surrounds you, which reflect the general state of health. Auric healers place their hands on or near the body and visualise healing colours to help the body to heal itself.

• Faith healing: Faith healers believe that without the patient's faith in their personal power of the deity or religious leader they represent, there can be no cure. Healing is usually performed in a religious setting often under circumstances of group activity and hysteria.

• Absent healing: healers aim to visualize a healing energy that they can send towards a receiver in far away.

Reiki

History

Reiki is an energy healing system based on ancient Tibetan knowledge it was re-discovered by a Japanese theologian in the mid 1800s by Mikao Usui, a Christian minister in Japan, who was challenged by his students to tell them how Jesus was able to heal. Dr Usui devoted many years of his life searching for the answer, and eventually after studying ancient Indian and Buddhist teachings, the roots of Reiki with its symbols and mantras were found.

It is one of the most ancient healing methods known to mankind, is a gentle yet very powerful method of healing body, mind and spirit. Reiki is a Japanese word in which the first syllable, Rei, means spirit, aura or subtle energy. The second syllable, Ki, means energy or power. In China it is called Qi and in India, Shakti or Prana. In English we use terms such as life-force, cosmic consciousness or divine energy.

Theory
Reiki practitioners transmit energy by a light touch, a gentle placing of hands in specific positions on the body. Reiki can be used for mental, emotional, physical, or spiritual balancing. Reiki practitioners are the first to say they don't exactly know how it works. There are a series of "attunements" or "empowerments" and most students only take the first and second-degree initiations, attunements that empower them to share energy in "hands-on sessions". Personal sessions can last one hour or longer. Reiki healing can also be sent over distances in the second stage of training, and it can be used on animals and plants. Reiki is a relaxing and meditative experience it can reduce tension and stress, treat many ailments and the symptoms and causes of insomnia. This natural method of healing works on many different levels balancing the energies in the body and it adapts to the natural needs of the receiver, whilst further enhancing personal awareness and intuition. Different people experience Reiki in different ways. The experience can range from feeling calm and centred to more energized, or both. Many other therapies, i.e. massage, aromatherapy and reflexology, also use Reiki as part of their treatments.

Treatment
Treatment will involve laying hands either on or just above the body in different positions or just above the persons head, this enables the healer to give the patient energy through

themselves to help to cure or restore the body or mind of the patient.

Relevance to insomnia
Reiki is very effective for insomnia, it relaxes and balances the body and is very calming.

Warning
Should not be done on any one with a pace maker or any one suffering from diabetes mellitus or appendicitis.

Reiki is quite safe for use with the terminally ill or dying and can be very calming, but should not be used solely in pathological conditions such as a broken leg but be used alongside traditional medicine to aid recovery.

Chapter 17

Hands on Therapies

Ayurvedic medicine

History

Ayurveda is a traditional medicine from India incorporating medicinal, psychological, cultural, religious, and philosophical concepts. Sometimes called the "mother of healing", Ayurveda means knowledge (ayur) and life (veda). Ayurvedic medicine is a practical "science of life", with principles for better health that can be applied to any individual's daily life. It was developed in India over the past 4,000 years, and covers all aspect of medicine. Ayurveda was discovered and developed by ancient Indian holy men known as "Rishis". Due to their link to both the spiritual and physical worlds, they were able to distinguish the fundamental nature of the universe and, thus, man's place in it. The goal of Ayurveda is true freedom from death and disease, enjoyment of everlasting physical, mental and spiritual happiness and fulfilment.

To early twentieth-century Westerners, Indian health practices seemed primarily to involve yoga and meditation and these were all but outlawed in India by the British colonial rule. In 1833, the East India Company closed and banned all Ayurvedic colleges, and for almost 100 years, Ayurveda was confined to the back streets of India. But after independence Ayurveda re-emerged and is now the most prominent form of practised medicine in India. Ayurveda has now been voted, by the World Health Organization (WHO), as the best hope for a base for global medicine in the undeveloped countries. This can be obtained by using localised herbs and remedies, adaptability to local conditions and customs combined with Western. Chinese and traditional native medicines blended in each locale.

Theory
Ayurveda works by removing the cause of the disease and keeps the body's immune system strong and able to combat everyday germs and ailments or to heal itself of chronic disorders including insomnia. Oriental medicines organize food, herbal remedies, and energies into five elements, Earth, Water, Fire, Air and Ether.

The Chinese divide the world and its material into yin and yang: the Indians into three bioforces: vata, pitta, and kapha (usually translated as wind, fire, and mucus).

As Tradition Chinese Medicine grew in strength and organization, it eventually overshadowed Ayurveda in China. But Ayurveda continued to develop and to become stronger in India. Good health, in Ayurvedic medicine, is a state of balance where one's body, mind, spirit, and environment are in harmony.

This harmony is achieved through the observation of proper diet, exercise, massage, and lifestyle habits, the practice of mediation and the maintenance of psychological wellness, especially through the tranquility that comes with self-acceptance and love.

Treatment
Ayurveda does not treat symptoms; it focuses on curing the cause of the disease. Diet which is tied to the power of digestion, is a primary consideration, eating the correct foods is essential and fasting one day a week is considered very beneficent ayurveda treatments can also include massage.

Many aspects of it can be used to support numerous treatment programmes, and it has been known to help skin problems, nausea, obesity, anxiety, digestive disorders, allergies, insomnia and many other ailments.

Relevance to insomnia
Ayurvedic medicine will help insomnia by putting the body back into balance and by treating the ailments that may be causing the sleep problems.

Warning
Should have no harmful side effects, but take care of essential oils used in the first few months of pregnancy.

Tibetan Medicine

History
Tibetan Medicine is a synthesis of Ayurvedic, Chinese and Greco-Persian medicine using acupuncture, herbalism, yoga, mediation and the Buddhist understanding of the mind/body relationship.

Theory
Tibetan herbal medicine, like that of India, seeks balance between three humours, bile, wind and phlegm. Once again each herb is categorized according to its taste, and also according to its relationship to the three elements. They believe the universe to be composed of five constituents, earth, water, fire, air and space. Bile has the nature of fire, phlegm the nature of earth, water and wind the nature of movement.

Treatment
Treatment can include diet, herbals and a change of life style; it will look at the contributory factors to the condition.

Relevance to insomnia
As with Ayurvedic medicine Tibetan medicine will help balance the system.

Warning
No known side effects.

Shiatsu

History
Shiatsu developed at the turn of the twentieth century from anma, as part of traditional Japanese medicine that has existed for 2000 years and it uses Oriental Medicine as its theoretical framework like Acupuncture and Acupressure. Originally used to treat very specific conditions, it has now developed as an aid to relaxation. The government of Japan recognized Shiatsu as an important and an effective therapy and it is now very poplar in Japan, Europe and the USA.

Theory
Shiatsu is a Japanese word, which literally translated means 'finger pressure'. But the techniques involve the use not only of fingers, but also thumbs, palms, knees, forearms, elbows and feet. Pressure is put on the tsubo points one the body, these tsubo (pressure points) run along the meridian lines that run the through the length of our bodies from head to toe. Physically this has the effect of stimulating the circulation and the flow of lymphatic fluid, working on both divisions of the autonomic nervous system, helping to release toxins and deep seated tension from the muscles and stimulating the endocrine (hormone) system.

Treatment
Shiatsu is a physical therapy applied at floor level by the therapist. Shiatsu works by stimulating the body's vital energy flow (known as Ki in Japanese) in order to promote

good health. Shiatsu treatments are given to you clothed in loose attire, a cotton jog suit is best, and they would take place on a padded mat on the floor.

Relevance to insomnia

Insomnia can be a by-product of many physical and psychological disorders. Oriental Medicine sees it as a deficiency of Heart energy and Blood, due to emotional problems or an unbalanced lifestyle. The Heart-Ki and Blood keep the Mind anchored and calm. Therefore, deficiency in either will cause the mind to be over active. This will be exacerbated at night if the body's cooling functions are weak (expressed as Yin deficiency in Oriental Medicine). Feeling too hot at night, with a restless mind, thus amounts to insomnia. A congested Liver may also cause sleeplessness. Shiatsu treatment similar to that given for depression may help, using pressure points that would work on the heart channel to calm the mind. If a congested Liver causes sleeplessness, dispersal of the Liver Channel will be given. Shiatsu, acupuncture and acupressure combined with Chinese herbs can be very successful for insomnia.

Warning

Not always suitable for older people, those with brittle bones or women in the first three months of pregnancy.

Reflexology

History

Reflexology is a method for activating the healing powers of the body; it is both old and new. From ancient texts, we know that the early Chinese, Japanese, and Egyptians worked on the feet to promote good health. What joins the ancients with the moderns is the principle that there are energy zones that run throughout the body and reflex areas in the feet, hands and ears that correspond to all the major organs, glands, and body parts. In the early years of the twentieth century, Dr William Fitzgerald developed the modern zone theory of the human body. He contended that parts of the body correspond to reflected areas in the feet and hands, and that applying pressure to one area anesthetized a corresponding area.

Theory
Reflexology yields the best results when the therapists work with dedication, patience and loving care. Reflexology reduces stress and induces deep relaxation; many clients fall asleep during a treatment and rise refreshed and relaxed. Reflexology has many benefits it helps the body to revitalise it self and to fight against disease. Reflexology is mainly practised on the feet but can also be done on hands and ears. The feet are remarkably sensitive and receptive, partly because of the wealth of nerve endings and partly because we keep them covered and protected.

Treatment
Treatments last about an hour, you will lie down on a couch or reclining chair with your feet slightly raised and the practitioner will work over all areas of the feet in a gentle kneading motion with his/her fingers and thumbs.

Relevance to insomnia
Reflexology is a very relaxing treatment and will often have you nodding off during a treatment; it will also help to balance your sleep system.

Warning
Treatment is not recommended for pregnant women, diabetics, epileptics or anyone receiving medical treatment or on medication except by a qualified therapist and with your doctor's permission. Most people feel relaxed after a treatment but some experience after effects such as: runny nose, thirst, light-headedness or wanting to go to the toilet. Children love having their feet massaged and find it very

calming and restful, but only use very gentle stroking movements when treating babies and young children.

Other information
Hand reflexology is an ideal alternative for elderly people, invalids, wheelchair bound or disabled and those that don't like having their feet touched. Massaging the reflexes of the ears can also help, headaches, tinnitus, and sleeplessness, and it is often included as one of the movements in Indian Head Massage.

Metamorphic Technique

History
An English naturopath, Robert St John, developed Metamorphic Technique after he studied reflexology. Reflexology works on the whole foot and on physical symptoms in the reflexology system the inner side of the foot, from the big toe to the heel, represents the head and spine.

Theory
St John discovered that this area also represents the period of conception and birth and by gently massaging it can release emotional traumas from that vital period of our life. Children can benefit enormously from the Metamorphic Technique, and often enjoy giving sessions to other people. A lot has been done to help children with Down's syndrome. The technique can also soothe children and adults who are suffering from birth trauma, or are hyperactive or highly-strung. Adult stroke patients, and people with nervous disorders can also benefit. The tensions and anxieties seem to drop away leading to relaxation and natural sleep.

Treatment
The technique is a very gentle form of massage of the feet, hands and head, but foremost, the feet. It is meant to

stimulate the receiver's powers of self-healing by releasing emotional blocks.

Relevance to insomnia
This technique is very relaxing; in fact it could have you nodding off during a session. It is designed to help you cope with problems, and clear out the stresses and tensions in the body that frequently cause insomnia.

Warning
It would be advisable to consult a doctor before treatment if there are any serious medical conditions or during pregnancy.

Inðían Heað Massage

History
Indian Head massage has its roots in the ancient medical system of Ayurveda and originated in India. It was initially practised in the home, and passed on from generation to generation, by Indian mothers to their children. For centuries Indian women have been keeping their long hair in good condition by massaging their heads with natural oils and stimulating blood flow to the hair follicles. The actions have the side effect of easing tension and leaving the recipient feeling wonderfully relaxed, making it the ideal therapy for headaches and insomnia. Head massage is part of the way of life for everyone in India, men will go to the barbers for a shave and to have a relaxing head massage, barbers finished off a haircut with 'champi' (head massage) from which our word shampoo is derived. Massage is part of the Indian way of life and you will find people offering Indian Head massage on the streets in Bombay and on the beaches of Goa.

Theory
Indian Head massage works by massaging the shoulders, neck, head and face with relaxing and stimulating strokes

and applying pressure with fingers and thumbs to the pressure points that help revitalize the scalp, face and hair and relieve tension and stress in the body. Most tension accumulates in the shoulders and neck, and Indian Head Massage stimulates blood flow through these areas to the head to release this tension.

Treatment
Indian head massage can be done while you are lying down or sitting up in a chair. It has been changed slightly for the western clients and now includes a back, neck, shoulder, head and face massage, usually with fragrant oils. It is calming and relaxing and good for relieving stress, headaches, sleeplessness and improving the condition of face and hair.

Relevance to insomnia
Indian Head massage is very relaxing, people often fall asleep during a treatment, it also helps with headaches and tension in the neck and shoulders that can cause sleep problems.

Warning
Consult a doctor if you have any serious medical condition, do not use essential oils during pregnancy and with certain medical conditions.

Thai Massage

History
Traditional Thai Massage can look back at a long history of therapeutic healing. If one traces the evolution of the techniques of Thai massage and healing the roots go back to India. To a doctor from Northern India known as Jivaka Kumar Bhaccha, who was a contemporary of the Buddha.

Theory
In Thailand the theoretical foundation of Thai massage is based on the concept of energy lines running through the body. Ten of these lines are especially important in Thai massage, massage these points, and it is claimed, it makes it possible to treat certain diseases or to relieve pain. Working on the energy lines with massage can break the blockages, stimulate the flow of energy and help to restore general well being.

Treatment
Thai massage differs from Swedish massage, which is the most widespread technique of massage in the West. The kneading of muscles, which dominates in Swedish massage, is absent from Thai. The therapist uses hands, feet and elbows to apply pressure to important points along these lines in combination with yoga based stretches. The treatment is both relaxing and energising. The yoga positions make it ideal for sports people and dancers, the blocking of energy lines in the body will aid restful sleep, and the energy line work out is especially beneficial during pregnancy and after giving birth.

Relevance to insomnia
Thai massage will help insomnia is it is a build up of tension in the body that is causing the sleep problems.

Warning
Not suitable for some pregnant women, elderly and people with brittle bone conditions, always consult a doctor if you have and any serious illness.

Rosen Method

History
The Rosen Method grew out of the studies and work of a refugee from Nazi Germany in the years after World War 11.

Marion Rosen was born in Nuremberg in 1914, as a young woman she studied relaxation techniques and massage and was a student on Carl Jung working on talk therapy. Jung's ex wife was a masseuse and dancer and did bodywork therapies, together they worked with dancers and combined massage, verbal expression and breathing sessions. Rosen later moved to America via Sweden and set up in San Francisco during the last years of the war as a therapist using what was then called the Rosen Method. In the 1970s she took on her first apprentices, and in 1980 she began her first professional training. Rosen Method is now practiced in many countries around the world.

Theory
Rosen Method bodywork combines touch and verbal contact to evoke muscular relaxation. Using light to medium touch to increase body self-awareness, this bodywork focuses on muscular tension, and the relationship between that tension and the emotions.

The role of breath is used in creating more space and flexibility in one's physical structure. Tension keeps the muscles unnecessarily contracted, inhibiting feelings and emotional expression. We are often taught as children to hold on to our emotions, for example 'boys don't cry, don't be a baby, control yourself'. We hide our feelings inside often leading to tight shoulders, stiff necks, headaches, insomnia and repressed feelings.

Treatment
Sessions are one hour and the practitioner uses gentle but forceful touch and supportive words. Rosen therapy involves breathing, massage, gentle range-of-motion exercises set to music, allowing the body to give up its tension and achieve its own natural awareness,

Relevance to insomnia

Rosen therapy allows emotions to come out, releasing the tension and stress being held in the body allowing the tension to leave our bodies, filling our lungs with air, and releasing our feelings of frustration and stress. The releasing and relaxing effects of this method are good for the body's immune system, circulation problems, fatigue, stress and insomnia.

Warning

(Rosen method works well with psychotherapy see page 161) Great care should by exercised when releasing old trauma and hidden feelings Rosen techniques works best when combined with other therapies that can help with the emerging trauma that can manifest in physical pain or emotional upset. Caution should be taken with pregnant women and those with chronic illness consult a doctor before treatment.

Stomach Rub

History

Stomach rub comes out of the general body works disciplines such as Aromatherapy and Ayurvedic medicine.

Theory

The massage of the stomach is very relaxing, it sooths down the digestive system and helps to bring about a deeper relaxation. An extra benefit is that it will help you to lose weight by improving the functioning of the digestive system and easing constipation.

Treatment

Simply lie on your back and place your hand on your navel, and begin to make small circles in a clockwise direction as you gently glide your hand over your stomach. Let your circles gradually become bigger and bigger, when your circles reach the outside of your stomach, gradually reduce their size until you are back at your navel again. Then reverse the direction and do the same thing over again. Repeat this whole series with your other hand adjusting the pressure to what is comfortable for you. If you can get someone else to do the tummy rub, so much the better, you can also use aromatherapy oils to aid digestion or for period pain. (see aromatherapy recipes on pages 189-190)

Relevance to insomnia
Having your tummy rubbed or rubbing it yourself is very relaxing and calming and can help induce restful sleep if performed last thing at night or lying in bed just before going to sleep.

Additional Information
Tummy rub can be included in treatments such as massage, aromatherapy and manual lymphatic drainage.

Warning
Foods moves through the colon in a clockwise direction and if you have trouble with constipation make all your circles clockwise. Take care if there may be a hernia or any other disorder or growth in this area.

Massage

History
Massage comes from the Greek '*masso*' to knead, and the Arabic '*mass*', to press gently. The term massage is sometimes used interchangeably with words such as bodywork, body therapies, and body manipulation. Technically, there are many different types of body therapies, manipulation therapies focus on restructuring the body, Osteopathy, Chiropractic, Alexander Technique, Rolfing and Postural Integration.

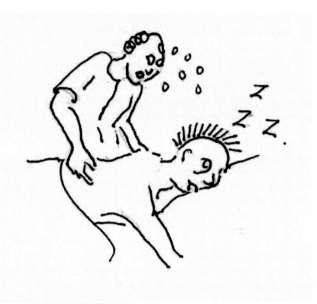

Massage is a healing art that is sensual, when practiced between lovers, it can be sexual and it can be difficult for some people to get away from the stigma of the 'massage parlor'. There are many styles of massage, many names from which to chose. The following form the wide-ranging kinds of massage available today:

• Swedish: the original health spa and sports club massage, uses a set routine of basic strokes to work over the whole body.

• Esalen: a blend of Eastern and Western approaches, primarily Swedish and acupressure; stress empathy, communication, and nurturance above the technique.

MLD or (Manual Lymphatic Drainage) encompasses several styles, it focuses on stimulating the lymphatic system, internal organs such as the liver, kidney, or colon, to flush toxins and mucus out of the body.

• Lomi: based on a Hawaiian Kahuna tradition; works deep tissue.

• Amma: based on ancient Oriental traditions that gave birth to Shiatsu and Kahuna energy-based massage; works tsubos, or energy points, stroking away from the heart.

• Subtle Touch: infuses touch with inspiration; reaches into muscle tension to contact and melt away painful emotional holdings.

• Sports Massage: used as part of athletic training; focuses specifically on muscle recovery rate to alleviate the aches and pains of exertion and competition.

• Rehabilitate or Medical massage: developed for post-World War 11 amputees and other wounded veterans; focuses on relieving pain from neurologic problems.

• Neuromuscular massage: This technique involves treatment of soft tissue lesions such as congestion's, nodules and knots with deep pressure movements.

• Indian Head massage: deep massage to the pressure points in the back, shoulders, arms, neck, head and face, incorporating many Swedish massage techniques.

• Aromatherapy massage: a gentler all over massage utilizing blended essential oils to create a very individual soothing

Theory
A massage session can sedate or stimulate the body, depending on the nature or style of strokes applied; a calming massage will relieve tension and relax body, mind and senses.

Treatment
The therapist will always take a detail consultation about general health and lifestyle. Treatments will vary according to different specialist kind of massage see under over headings i.e. Aromatherapy and Indian Head Massage. Most treat-ments are given on a massage couch, but treatment can be adapted to a chair, floor or bed as circumstances necessitate. Therapeutic masseurs and masseuses usually use oil, but can also use talc or cream, the client or patient is unclothed and draped with sheets or towels.

Relevance to insomnia
For insomnia sufferers a soothing massage at bedtime undoubtedly promotes sleep, the result can not only certain but prompt. Massage has the advantage over all kinds of narcotics that there are no dangerous side effects. Massage becomes more effective the more often it is used, and gives a deep natural sleep without after-effects in the morning.

Warning
Always inform your doctor if you have any medical condition and you are having massage or any other complementary therapy, for example massage is not always recommended if you suffer from diabetes.

Other information
Find an all-round qualified massage therapist, and possibly take yourself and your partner or a friend and go to a class and learn yourself, you will never regret it.

Children and babies often love to be massaged, and it can be a marvelous bonding tool between parents and babies.

Chapter 18

Aromatherapy

Aromatherapy

History
Aromatherapy is a multifaceted healing art, which uses the essential oils of aromatic plants and trees to promote health of body and serenity of mind. The history of the application of essential oils to the human body goes back at least 4000 years. The Greeks and Romans used perfumed oils for scented massage and in daily baths. They discovered that the odour of certain plants and flowers was stimulating and invigorating, while others were sedative and relaxing. Hippocrates, a Greek physician, wrote about a vast range of medicinal plants, and claimed that the best way to achieve good health and restful sleep was to have an aromatic bath and scented massage every day! The earliest written record of the use of aromatic oils in England was in the 13th century.

It is a known fact that people who used aromatic oils were the only ones to survive the Plague. The knowledge of the medicinal properties of plants was later reinforced by Nicholas Culpeper, a celebrated herbalist who wrote a book of herbs in 1652 which contained the medicinal properties of hundred of plants.

Treatment
Aromatherapy massage is a wonderful way to relax, a qualified therapist should ideally do it, but great benefits can be had by massage from a partner or sympathetic friend. But a well-trained therapist will tune into your needs and individually create the right blend of oils specifically for you.

Relevance to insomnia
Aromatherapy can be an invaluable aid in all its many forms in the assistance to promoting restful sleep. The olfactory nerves in the nose lead to the limbic or emotional centre of the brain, and certain smells have a calming effect and can help calm the mind in preparation for sleep.

Warning
Never use more than 8 drops of any essential to a bath of water or 5 drops of essential to a 5 ml of oil for massage, for a child 3 or 4 drops of any oil will be enough (see chart on page 188) Essential oils must never be taken internally, and you should never put full-strength essential oils directly on to the skin, the only oils you can use neat on to the skin are Tea Tree and Lavender. Trust your own nose, if you don't like the smell it is very doubtful that it will do you any good.

Always keep essential oils away from the sexual organs it will cause irritation because the penis and vagina would to be too sensitive. Nursing mothers must also be aware that a baby suckling on a breast could imbibe any residues of oil left on the breast, be sure to clean this area carefully before breast feeding. Some essential oils are not suitable for pregnant women or nursing mothers, see portraitures of essential oils below. Clary Sage is a relaxant, which should never be combined with alcohol, as the two together can induce very strong dreams. Always treat aromatherapy oils with respect, always take great care when buying and using essential oils and purchase them from a reputable supplier.

186

Additional information
Breathing aromatic vapours in the bedroom helps to induce sleep: Frankincense is warming and relaxing, and encourages tranquility. Marjoram has excellent soporific properties and dabbing two drops on the edge of your pillow can harness Lavender's relaxing quality. Release essential oils in a light-bulb ring or fragrancer. Neroli's wonderful floral fragrance is also seductive; two drops on the pillow or in a fragrancer will help disperse unpleasant thoughts. Baths before bedtime with lavender, rose and camomile oil really helps you to relax. Bergamot is a good choice where insomnia is linked with depression.

Try a gentle hand and foot massage before going to bed, use 5 ml of Sweet Almond or Sesame oil with 5 drops of Lavender, Marjoram, Frankincense or Rose essential oil. A hot footbath before bed also helps relaxation you can use 4 drops Peppermint or Lavender oil to relieve tired feet.

Essential Oils for Babies and Children
There are many different essential oils, not all of which are suitable or entirely safe for pregnant women, babies and children. For newborn babies only a handful of essential oils are recommended, but you can add other essences as the child grows, providing certain precautions are observed. Children can respond very well to aromatherapy and all natural forms of healing. This could be because they do not have the prejudices of some older people or because their young bodies have excellent powers of recuperation. Their forces of self-healing have not, hopefully, yet been damaged by years of faulty diet, stress, unhealthy lifestyle, and environmental pollution.

For babies and young children choose just one of the essences recommended below at a dilution of 1 to 3 drops per 30 ml base oil. For children over 6 years old you can make simple blends of two different essential oils at a dilution of 6 to 10 drops per 30 ml of base oil. Never use essential oils undiluted (with the exception of very small amounts of lavender or tea tree on burns, spots or insect bites). Always dilute essential oils before adding them to a bath for a child and use less oil, not more that 4 drops for a child in an average size bath. Stop using immediately, any oil that the child dislikes the smell of, or has an adverse skin reaction to. The use of the following oils should be avoided before going out into the sun or using a sun bed: Bergamot, cedarwood, ginger, patchouli, and all citrus oils, (lemon, grapefruit, mandarin ect). It is advisable to regulate the frequency with which you use essential oils, for example do not use the same oil continuously for a long period, but rotate different oils. It is advisable to avoid all essential oils in the first three months of pregnancy and if there is any history of miscarriage. Always seek professional advice and if in any doubt do not use any essential oils during pregnancy.

Oils to use for babies and children

Newborn babies	Camomile, lavender, fennel,
2 to 6 months	As above plus grapefruit, geranium, sweet orange, mandarin.
6 to 12 months	As above plus eucalyptus, and tea tree.
1 to 5 years	As above plus peppermint.
5 to 7 years	As above plus patchouli, black pepper, marjoram, rosemary, sandalwood, niaouli, lemon and ginger.

| Over 7 years | As above plus frankincense, melissa, basil, rose, bergamot. |

Recípes foR aRomatheRapy

Try some of the following blends, buy a good aromatherapy book (see recommended book list) and experiment with your own combinations. But always take care to follow safety rules when using essential oils. The vast majority of essential oils are perfectly safe for home use, provided they are used correctly. Judiciously applied they can help to enhance mood, promote relaxation, and relieve some ailments. But the user must be aware that essential oils are highly concentrated plant extracts, which can be 99 times as strong as oils occurring naturally in plants.

<u>Massage</u> <u>blends</u>　　　　　　　**<u>for</u> <u>bath</u> <u>or</u> <u>burner</u>**

For depression leading to inability to sleep

30ml sweet almond oil	4 drops ylang ylang
6 drops of lavender	4 drops lavender
6 drops of geranium	4 drops ylang ylang

For restless legs syndrome at night

30ml sweet almond	4drops bergamot
5 drops camomile (Roman)	4drops camomile (Roman)
4 drops bergamot	
5 drops lavender	

For restlessness and too active brain keeping you awake

30ml sweet almond	
5 drops frankincense	4 drops frankincense
5 drops lavender	4 drops lavender
5 drops grapefruit	

For winter blues (SAD)

30ml sweet almond

5 drops grapefruit

5 drops lavender

2 drops rose

4 drops grapefruit

4 drops lavender

For painful memories and worries that are stopping you sleep

30ml Sweet almond

5 drops frankincense

5 drops grapefruit

2 drops neroli

8 drops frankincense

Insomnia disturbed sleep and nightmares

30ml sweet almond

5 drops lavender

5 drops camomile (Roman)

5 drops mandarin

3 drops lavender

3 drops camomile (Roman)

3 drops mandarin

Lying awake with worry or anxiety

30ml sweet almond

5 drops camomile (Roman)

5 drops sandalwood

4 drops lemon

5 drops camomile (Roman)

2 drops lemon

3 drops lavender

Relaxing Colour Bath

Run a bath before bed time and put a few drops of blue or green vegetable colour into the running water then when the bath is full put 10 drops of lavender essential oil into the water and stir with your hands. Relax in the bath for 15 minutes and then prepare for bed.

Essential oils are highly volatile and flammable, so keep them away from heat, sunlight and naked flames, always store in a safe, cool dark place away from children.

Chapter 19
Other Techniques

Rolfing

History
In the 1060's Ida P Rolf called her system Structural
Integration, which described her original goal in creating it.
Due to family illness some thirty years earlier she investigated the causes of poor posture and came to the conclusion
that poor posture put the body out of balance physically and
emotionally.

The object of Rolfing is to increase muscular length and
overall balance for optimum posture, as measured along a
vertical axis from the ear to the ankle. An aligned body
balances better against gravity, allowing the body to use
energy more efficiently.

Rolfing Movement Integration applies new postural
consciousness to every day action. Rolf explored the ideas of
the Alexander Technique and studied osteopathy
incorporating the view that structure determines function. If
the body were out of balance it would constrict its physical
and mental functioning.

Theory
The free flow of energy aids the body's own ability to heal
itself, this is a principle stated over and over again in many

different ways, by healing arts from Traditional Chinese Medicine, Shiatsu, Reflexology, Acupuncture and Acupressure to Polarity Therapy. Rolf saw the body as a group of stackable units, structured by bones and soft tissue, bones hold the body's position in space, and soft tissues, muscles, tendons and ligaments hold the bones in position. If muscles are shortened, they pull the attached bones out of balance.

Treatment
Rolfing is a series of ten hour-long bodywork sessions of deep connective tissue manipulation to balance the distribution of weight of the major parts of the body by stretching and lengthening soft tissues, when the line is straight, the body can move with more grace and efficiency.

A Rolfing session will begin with a medical history, and measurements of the body against a plumb line from ear to ankle. The sessions will contain breathing, and body manipulations; it can at times be uncomfortable or even painful. Most people who come to be rolfed will be uncomfortable in their bodies, i.e. have hunched shoulders, or be in physical pain in some way.

Relevance to insomnia
It can help insomnia suffers if there is pain and discomfort, or getting comfortable in bed is the reason for sleeplessness.

Warning
Rolfing may not always be suitable; persons with cancer, emotional trauma, brittle bones and acute conditions such as osteoporosis should avoid Rolfing. It may also not be appropriate for people who bruise very easily or people who are obese.

Alexander Technique

History
Frederick Matthias Alexander was born in Australia, he was sickly and premature and not expected to live. He was plagued with one illness after another, mainly asthma and other respiratory difficulties. His childhood health difficulties continued into adulthood until he developed his own techniques to combat them. It was his conviction that we suffer from headaches, backache, arthritis, insomnia, and many other ailments because of incorrect alignment in our body. He later became an actor and was able to help develop his voice and posture, as well as help many others in that profession.

Theory
This bad posture and tension in our bodies causes lack of coordination and balance and interferes with other reflexes throughout the body. The Alexander Technique is not so much a therapy but a education on how to hold your body, the teacher helps the patient develop an awareness of there body, posture, and postural bad habits. Many of these bad habits are carried through from childhood and a good posture is something that has to be relearned, it can effect all the functions of the body; breathing, circulation, digestion and bowel movements and sleeping.

Treatment
After an initial consultation about general health and lifestyle, it will be very relevant what work you do and any sports of hobbies you partake in. The teacher will then ask you to walk around the room and sit down, to see how you use your body.

Having observed your posture and how you move the teacher may then ask you to lie on a couch, with our head raised on a block or a pile of books and your knees raised, while he/she uses his/her hands to relax your muscles and re-align your limbs. You would wear loose garments that will enable you to move easily and allow the teacher to observe your body movements.

Relevance to insomnia
Insomnia is often caused by anxiety in some form, by practising Alexander Technique you can release much of the tension that has built up over the years and this in turn helps you to feel calmer and able to sleep better. Practising specific movements and exercises to get the body back into a relaxed alignment does this.

Warning
Alexander technique has no harmful effects if taught by a qualified practitioner and is suitable for all ages.

Chiropractic

History
Chiropractic is the Western world's third largest primary health care profession, after medicine and dentistry. The name comes from the Greek words *chiro* and *prakrikos*, meaning "done by hand". Chiropractic was developed by a Canadian osteopath, David Daniel Palmer in 1895. Palmer later set up the Palmer Infirmary and Chiropractic Institute in Iowa, USA. The practice of chiropractic has grown rapidly and there are about 50,000 practitioners in the USA. In the UK there are now well over 1,000 chiropractors and the therapy is recognised in medical circles.

Theory
A Chiropractor will manipulate the skeletal muscular system of the body, usually by hand. The aim is adjustment of the spinal column to restore normal nervous system functioning.

The scope of chiropractic practice ranges from the traditional, which stick mainly to spinal manipulation, to the more popular liberal view that view chiropractic as enveloping every health care tool except drugs and surgery.

Treatment
It is necessary to take a full and detailed consultation of general health and lifestyle. The practitioner will then observe the client walking and moving to evaluate the extent of the problem. Treatment then comprises gentle manipulation of the spine using the hands, fingers and elbows but can include soft tissue work to stretch muscles and connective tissue and relax the body. It may be necessary to get an X-ray and other standard medical tests to investigate any underlying disease and you may be referred back to your GP.

Relevance to insomnia
Chiropractic therapy will certainly help where stress, body discomfort and pain is inhibiting sleep.

Warning
Chiropractic is not suitable for broken bones, trapped nerves or people with osteoporosis.

Osteopathy

History
The science, of osteopathy, which was developed prior to the creation of chiropractic, is now practised side by side with orthodox medicine. An American doctor and trained engineer, Andrew Taylor Still, founded osteopathy in the 1870s. The name 'osteopathy' from the Greek words *osteo* (meaning bone) and *pathos* (meaning disease). The therapy came over to the UK at the beginning of the twentieth century and a school was set up on London in 1917.

Theory
Like the other manipulative therapies, it focused on keeping the body in structural balance so it can heal itself. However, an osteopath may medicate with prescription drugs as well as herbal substances and treat serious or infectious diseases and will work alongside the orthodox medical practitioner. Osteopaths both diagnose problems and treat the whole person by manipulating the muscular-skeletal system, with massage and manipulation.

Treatment
The therapist will ask about your medical and life history in a full consultation that can take up most of the first session. Treatment comprises massage and manipulation of the joints of the body; the therapist will ask you do a range of movements to assess your mobility.

Relevance to insomnia
As with chiropractic therapy it will help where the body is in pain or discomfort (particularly back pain) and this is stopping you from sleeping it can also help with emotional trauma and tension.

Warning
Not suitable for people with osteoporosis, rheumatoid arthritis, pregnancy (during the first three months), recent fractures and whiplash injuries.

Kinesiology

History
The system was founded in the 1960s by an American chiropractor, Dr George Goodheart. He found that some muscles appeared to be weak because there was sluggishness in the system and by massaging specific reflex points, the muscles would strengthen. Dr Goodheart developed a series of

muscle tests based on the muscle/meridian connection. Instead of using acupuncture he used gentle touch to the various muscles and that these muscles corresponded with organs and different parts of the body.

Theory
Kinesiology uses gentle muscle testing to 'communicate' with a person at the body level; the body level is where the records are stored. It can be a very effective way to find where a problem lies, or for detecting food allergies. It then endeavours to correct those imbalances by using various techniques. These may involve the simple rubbing of reflex points on the trunk, or holding points on the head, to strengthen a muscle/meridian association. Applied Kinesiology features pressure point and manipulative techniques, based on Chinese medicine's acupuncture theory, and employs neurolymphatic and neurovascular reflexes as they relate to structural, chemical, and mental physiology regulating mechanisms.

Treatment
The therapist will take a full consultation and do some muscle tests using gentle massage and manipulation of the muscles of the body and some practitioners may use magnets, gems, and colour to help with allergy testing. Kinesiology is often used to identify allergies and sensitivity to certain foods.

Relevance to insomnia
The effectiveness for insomnia sufferers will depend on the underlying problem or reason for the insomnia, but can be a good diagnostic tool in discovering why you are having sleep problems.

Warning
No side effects but take if you have any recent scars or varicose veins these may be uncomfortable under pressure or massage.

Traditional Chinese Herbal Medicine

History
Chinese medicine, part of traditional Chinese medicine, has been practised for over 5,000 years. The father of Chinese herbal medicine is thought to be the Emperor Yen (Shen Nong, c 1500 BC), who experimented with herbs and compiled a comprehensive list of herbal remedies and cures for many ailments. This has been added to over the years and today many volumes of books exist listing thousands of herbals.

Theory
Chinese medicine is not just a question of knowing where to insert needles or which herbs to brew. A Chinese doctor will look at the complete physiological and psychological profile of the individual, of which the symptom is merely a factor, to find the disharmony. The disease is a result of an imbalance in the flow of Qi through the body, and a strong element of Chinese health care such as Tai Chi is dedicated to precluding this imbalance.

Qi originally meant air, breath or energy, and then came to mean the vital nourishing and protecting energy. Animating Qi is a constant movement of energy between two opposing but complementary forces, each is said to be necessary for the other, and when one dominates, disease and emotional instability will follow. A number of factors can upset the delicate balance of yin and yang: infections, poisons and accidents or trauma; emotional states such as stress, anger or grief, spiritual neglect; inadequate or wrong diet, and drugs.

Treatment
Practitioners believe that by correcting the vital energy and Xue (blood) you can clear any blockage that is upsetting the balance and harmony of the body. Practitioners will look at the patient's lifestyle, including exercise and nutrition, and will recommend a healthy, whole food diet. Medicines will

have one of five flavours (pungent, sour, sweet, bitter, or salty), five Qi attributes (hot, cold, warm, cool or neutral) and four directions (ascending, floating, descending or sinking). The combination of these properties gives a herb/herbs a particular attribute.

Relevance to insomnia

For insomnia the Chinese herbalist will want to find out what is contributing to the lack of sleep. Chinese medicine also states that too much sleep is as unhealthy as too little and that both problems are a sign of imbalance. In Chinese medicine waking frequently is due to a deficiency of yin energy, which can be caused by overwork, stress, emotional strain, and poor diet. Chinese medical practitioners see yin deficiency as a common cause of insomnia in the elderly.

Warning

Be very careful when choosing a practitioner, some remedies may contain products from animals, some of which may be endangered species.

Acupuncture

History

Acupuncture is a Chinese method of treatment using needles that goes back thousands of years. Cave painting in China depict what looks like acupuncture needles on their walls. Missionaries brought acupuncture to Europe in the nineteenth century and other people retuning form the colonies. French diplomat, Georges Soulie de Morant who had worked in China in the 1930's published an acupuncture manual called *A Summary of the True Art of Chinese Acupuncture*. Acupuncture is now an excepted part of every day medicine and is used in operations as well as for treating many ailments.

Theory

One explanation of how acupuncture works is that a nerve impulse is fired off to the spinal cord from the needle insertion. This in turn releases the body's natural pain killer, endorphin. Endorphin is most abundant in a zone of the spinal cord concerned with sensation and appears to modify the sensation of pain. The pain-killing action of opium narcotics such as morphine maybe due to their imitating the natural effect of endorphins, to which they are chemically related.

Some people also believe that acupuncture causes the release of three neurotransmitters in the brain, which have the effect of making you feel drowsy and relaxed and have an impact on the body's hormones, which in turn can have a beneficial effect. It is also thought to influence the limbic centre in the brain that controls mood and behaviour.

Treatment

Your first session will consist of a detailed consultation in which you will relate any health problems and give details of your lifestyle. During an Acupuncture session you will lie prone on a couch and the therapist will insert needles into your body at specific points along the meridian lines.

In a recent development, some doctors use a very weak electrical current to stimulate the needles in the acupuncture points, instead of twisting the needles as in the traditional method

Relevance to insomnia

Acupuncture has often been used for pain relief; however, it can be used to treat almost anything that you would go to your GP for, including back pain, migraine, menopausal symptoms, and insomnia.

Warning
It should never be necessary to draw blood or to bleed in anyway during an acupuncture treatment. Do not partake in any alternative treatment that requires the taking of blood, unless under the supervision of your doctor or hospital.

Acupressure

History
Acupressure dates back thousands of years and comes out of the Chinese traditions of acupuncture; it can also be compared to the disciplines of shiatsu. Acupressure uses the same pressure points as acupuncture but instead of needles uses the gently but firm pressure of the hands and feet.

Theory
Acupressure is an ancient healing art that uses the fingers to press key points on the surface of the skin to stimulate the body's natural self-curative abilities. When these points are pressed, they release muscular tension and promote the circulation of blood and the body's life force to aid healing. Acupuncture and acupressure use the same points, but acupressure does not use needles.

Treatment
According to traditional Chinese medicine, an uneven distribution of energy can cause insomnia. In such cases, certain meridians (the energy pathways that connect acupressure points) become overloaded, while others become blocked. By pressing certain points, you can correct this energy imbalance.

Relevance to insomnia
Acupressure can be very helpful in relieving insomnia it is a relaxing treatment an ideal for stress related conditions.

Warning
Care should be taken with varicose veins, brittle bones and tender skin conditions, but otherwise acupressure is a safe therapy suitable for all ages.

Other information
There are acupressure points on the heel that have been used for relieving and preventing insomnia. The point on the inside of the heel is called Joyful Sleep; the one on the outside of the heel is called Calm Sleep. Massaging and pressing these points together on both sides of the heel enables the body to relax deeply and promote sleep. According to Chinese health care, insomnia is also related to the heart and pericardium meridians. If you have a blockage in either of these meridians, you may have difficulty sleeping. There are points of the wrist called Spirits Gate located on the inside of the wrist, below the little finger, and Inner gate Located on the centre of the wrist, two finger's widths above the wrist crease that are used for insomnia. These points help balance and calm the heart and alleviate anxiety.

Natural Reconnective Therapy

History
With origins in Egypt this therapy uses gentle pressure of different points of the body, it is like a deep relaxing massage concentrating on the connective tissue.

Theory
The theory is that the body contains memory banks, where specific tensions are stored. For example, the heart memory bank and the nervous system memory bank can be found in the shoulder blades. So part of the treatment would be to massage those areas and eliminate the stress held there. By treating the nervous system memory can erase the effects of emotional trauma and stress, which deprive so many people of

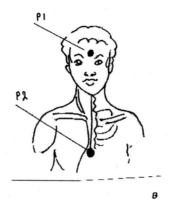

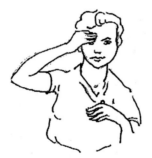

P1 Third Eye Position
Location: Between the eyebrows above the bridge of the nose. This position relieves anxiety.

P2 Breast Bone Position
Location: On the centre of the breastbone three thumb widths up from the base of the bone. This position relieves nervousness, chest congestion and the anxiety that causes insomnia.

Place the fingertips of your right hand on P1 and the fingertips of your left hand on P2. Close your eyes and breathe deeply for one minute.

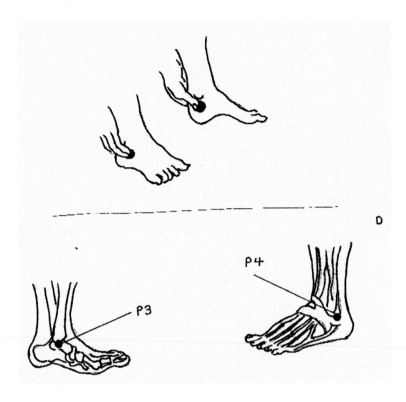

P3 Blissful Sleep
Location: Directly below the inside of the anklebone in a slight indentation.

P4 Peaceful Sleep
Location: In the first indentation directly below the outer anklebone.

Both these positions relieve pain in the feet and legs and help calm the body for sleep. Use both your thumbs to hold the P points. Hold for one minute and breathe deeply.

e

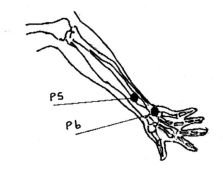

f

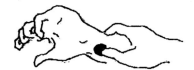

P5 Inner Wrist One
Location: In the middle of the inner side of the forearm, 21/2 finger
widths from the wrist crease. Relieves palpitations, nausea,
indigestion and insomnia due to anxiety.

P6 Inner Wrist Two
Location: On the inside of the wrist crease, in line with the little
finger. Relieves anxiety, cold sweats and insomnia due to
overexcitement.

Press these points individually with your thumb. Hold for one minute
breathing deeply.

sleep. The therapy will also maintain that you look at a problem as a whole, and recommend diet and relaxation.

Treatment
Practitioners use their thumbs to separate and realign the vertebrae, totally painlessly. Like many other natural therapies, it claims to restore the body's self-healing mechanisms, and it can treat not only difficult muscular and skeletal problems like whiplash injury and slipped discs, but also other conditions like insomnia.

Relevance to insomnia
It will help with sleeplessness, not by dealing with specific aches and pains but by erasing stress and tension from the body.

Warning
Not suitable for people with brittle bones or osteoporosis.

Cranio Sacral Massage and Cranial Osteopathy

History
Cranio sacral therapy is primarily concerned with creating a healthy balanced state on all levels, thereby eliminating disease and dysfunction. It can therefore help in almost any condition including insomnia, tinnitus, headaches, behavioural disorders, depression and ME. It is suitable for all ages, and as well as treating many specific conditions, it is also very effective at promoting general health and well-being and reintegrating following illness, accident or injury.

Theory
Cranial osteopathy is a gentle process of manipulating the bones of the skull and neck with such a light touch that many claim that they can barely feel it. It is based on the principle

that there is potential for movement in the joints between the fused bones of the head, and that compression or misalignment can cause health problems.

Cranio Sacral therapy is ideal for children; it treats the whole person, and all aspects of a person. It is not limited to the head or conditions affecting the head, although it does have a special role to play in the treatment of cranial compression due to Birth Trauma.

Treatment
Treatment involves a very light contact of the practitioner's hands on the client's cranium, sacrum or other appropriate part of the body, identifying subtle disturbances to the free motion of body tissues and the free flow of body fluids, which in turn reflect the underlying causes of ill health. The therapist will need to take a detailed history of the client's health and mental background including childhood trauma and emotional problems.

Relevance to insomnia
Cranial osteopathy practitioners recognise the intimate relationship between body and mind, that you cannot divorce the two. This therapy has had great success in treating headache, migraine and sleep problems that are related to the head like vertigo, tinnitus (ringing in the ears) and earache.

Warning
Considered safe in most circumstances.

Chapter 20

Other Complementary Therapies and Related Assistance

Photodynamic Therapy or Light Therapy

History
Light therapy has been developed for those suffering from SAD (see pg 133-134) and for some skin problems.

Theory
Light Therapy is a scientifically proved answer to many health problems including skin ailments such as acne and eczema. Studies with different types of depression have shown great improvement and good results have also been reported for helping people on shift work, or suffering from jet lag, depression, PMS and insomnia. Some lights act upon the circulation, some stimulate the production of serotonin a substance which helps with depression, and others help strengthen the skin, so helping with skin disorders and the aging process there is also some evidence that light treatments can help with some cancers.

Treatment
Using a light box or full spectrum lights can help in many ways, also try the natural alarm clock which increases light

gradually in the morning to stimulate the faint glimmer of dawn, gently getting brighter and brighter to light up the room until it reaches it's full intensity when a normal alarm beeper then sounds. The theory is that light governs the body clock, waking up to dawn provides a signal to body clock which keeps it synchronized. During winter, when most people have to wake before down, or for people who start work unusually early, the correct signal is not received and the internal 'circadian rhythms' are not in harmony. The natural alarm clock provides the missing signal. Our 'body clock' responds to this stimulus by speeding up and reinforcing the 'waking up process'. So that we have more or less woken up even before our eyes are open. This explanation probably goes back to when mankind was evolving, and our systems adapted so that our ancestors woke with the sunrise, which their bodily systems recognised as being a gradual increase in light.

Relevance to insomnia
Light therapy can really help for those in irregular sleep cycles and those who have problems getting up in the morning and sufferers of SAD. (For information on suppliers of melatonin and full spectrum lights and for information on light therapy practitioners see useful addresses in appendix 1)

Warning
Avoid long term exposure to ultra violet light as in will burn the skin.

Sleep With Your Head Facing North
Many groups of people have something to say about the direction you sleep in, but according to experts of geopathic stress we should sleep with our head facing north. This aligns your body with the electromagnetic field of the planet, bringing your own energies into harmony with those of the Earth.

Ionizers

There is increasing evidence that animals and plants thrive on air that is negatively charged. Negative ions act on our capacity to use oxygen, they increase the ability of the respiratory tract to deal with airborne allergens, dust and smoke particles. Histamine, which triggers hay fever, is dramatically reduced in level by negative ions, which also have a very beneficial effect on anyone suffering from bronchial complaints such as bronchitis, asthma, catarrh and colds. Work done in the University of California discovered that air ions act on the blood and brain levels of the hormone serotonin, a powerful and versatile hormone that induces deep neurovascular, endocrinal and metabolic effect. It is concerned with the transmission of nervous impulses and occurs in considerable quantities in the lower mid-brain, where it plays important roles in such basic patterns of life as sleep and our evaluation of moods. High levels of serotonin are associated with allergic reaction, eczema, lethargy, insomnia and depression.

Ionizers are electrical devises that emit negative ions that help to clear dust, smoke, and some allergens. Ions are positive and negative electrically charged molecules.

Positive ions contribute to restlessness, headaches, joint aches, respiratory problems and sleeplessness. Positive ions come from synthetic fabrics, pollution, dust, central heating, electrical appliances and smoking. In you living and working environment always try to keep a flow of fresh air, use natural products in furnishing where possible, do not smoke and avoid smoky environments and allow anyone to smoke in your bedroom.

Magnotherapy

History

The use of magnets goes back thousands of years, records show that the Egyptians, Greeks, Romans and ancient Indian cultures relied on magnetic therapy to treat and heal a wide range of ailments. Today, scientists, physicists and biologists agree that magnetism influences all forms of life, including human health. The earths magnetic field is created by electrical currents that flow within the liquid core of the planet just as human beings are electrical creatures all our major bodily functions are electrical. i.e. brain, heart and nerves. The magnetic fields of all living things can be disturbed by environmental pollution and radiation, chemical toxins, artificial fertilizers and pesticides reduce the vitamin and mineral contents of foods. Hormones and antibiotics are having less effect and superbugs (antibiotic resistant bacteria) are becoming more prevalent.

Theory

Magnet Therapy is based upon the principle that every organ in the body has its own vibrational) or oscillatory) rate, or frequency. Studies show that these frequencies can be disturbed by changes in out electromagnetic field, brought about by external factors, which in turn can result in a loss of well being and illness.

Treatment

The therapist will place suitable magnets on the body in close proximity to were disturbances exist, they create biochemical and metabolic changes within the body, thereby restoring each organ's vibrational frequency to it's natural harmonious level.

Relevance to insomnia

Because magnets can restore balance and they can treat pain and stress in the body they can help with insomnia.

Other information
Pain clinics regularly use magnets and many beauty
treatments include the use of magnets to delay the signs of
aging. Some companies do sell sleep kit's, which include
mattresses and pillows. You can also buy magnetic jewelry,
pads for placing on the body and to put in the bed or under
the pillow.

Warning
The magno-pads should not be used with those who have a
heart pacemaker fitted or have any metal plates in their body,
but are otherwise safe to use.

The Ozone Layer and the Etheric Field
The ozone layer that surrounds the Earth and protects all
living organisms within it could be described as the etheric
field of the earth's crust, similar to the etheric field or aura of
the human body. Ozone is a gas closely related to oxygen,
which helps to keep the Earth's atmosphere balanced and
thereby serves as a vital function to life.

Feng Shui

History
Feng Shui almost certainly grew out of the recognition that
man tends to prosper in certain environments, a balance of
heat and cold, colour and landscape.

Feng Shui is more than just a guide to arranging your home;
it is an ancient Chinese way of viewing the universe, deeply
bound up with Chinese astrology and the I Ching.

Theory
Feng Shui's guiding principle seeks to achieve harmony by
balancing the energies within the home and working

environment. It seeks to maximize positive energy and bring happiness and prosperity into the home, The position of the rooms in the house and the layout within those rooms play a vital role in determining the well-being and fortunes of the occupants

Treatment
A Feng Shui consultant will come to your home or work place and assess the layout, colours, and environmental stress in the area. They will then make recommendations for changes to all areas of your living space to make it more harmonious.

Relevance to insomnia
Feng Shui can help with insomnia if your bedroom environment is not conducive to sleep: the colour scheme may be wrong; the bed may be in the wrong place or the wrong room. Paying attention to the direction in which we sleep is one of the most important aspects of the layout of the bedroom. Many people have strong feelings about the direction in which they sleep, some finding one direction comfortable, and others finding the same direction uncomfortable and the noticeable cause of restless nights. It is said that Charles Dickens always had to sleep with his head pointing north and many believe that this is the best direction, the practice of Yoga would suggest east is best, in Feng Shui the best position can be worked out from your own special number and is often north/west for many people.

Warning
If employing a Feng Shui consultant make sure that they are properly qualified, ask to see references. If attempting to do it yourself, take it very slowly and don't make lots of changes in one go. Read lots of books and experiment before making major permanent changes.

Other Information
If practical it is sometimes handy just to experiment with sleeping directions, if only to confirm for oneself the basic validity of this belief. Objectively it has been established that the direction of the Earth's magnetic field definitely has an effect on the quality of sleep. The head of your bed should be pointed in one of your best directions, the bed direction can affect all sorts of things including career, but especially sleep, relationship and marriage luck.

There are a few basic rules of Feng Shui, which should not be broken:

• Try to sleep with the head of the bed placed against a wall for support as this reinforces your sense of security. Headboards likewise help with this feeling of support in the same way that a mountain range situated behind a house gives it support.

• The main one being that you should not sleep with your head pointed towards the door of the bedroom. This is because consciously or subconsciously there will always be a feeling of uneasiness about who might be entering the room if they cannot immediately be seen.

• Make sure you do not face the open door of an en-suit bathroom, as the stagnant water-produced ch'i from here will weaken your ch'i accumulation.

• Electric blankets, which cause you to sleep in a magnetic field, are to be avoided. If you must use them, then use them to warm the bed first, and then turn them off before getting into bed. If extra heat is needed it would be better to use a hot water bottle for an hour or so before retiring and then remove it when you get into bed.

• Mirrors should be placed where they cannot be seen from the bed. The same applies to mirror tiles because they 'break up' the image, and therefore the relationship reflected in them.

• Bedrooms should not be in a room with an open space underneath them, a storeroom or a garage; this creates a ch'i vacuum underneath and adversely affects the occupants. Also avoid sleeping in a room with an overhead beam, especially one that passes over the bed itself.

• As a basic rule you want to create a relaxing atmosphere with soft colours, no sharp corners and with restful pictures (to encourage love and loving relationships have pictures with happy loving couples in them) and comfortable furnishings.

• No electrical equipment should be in the bedroom, keep computers and televisions out of the bedroom if possible.

• Blue and gold are good colours for bedrooms, red accessories are good for love and passion and blues, mauves and purples to encourage restful sleep.

• Plants with round leaves can be beneficial as they help remove air pollutants, not too many though as they can remove oxygen at night.

• Lighting should be restful, bedside lights, subtle up lighters or concealed lighting is best, a dark room is easier to sleep in.

• Avoid clutter, keep your bedroom tidy, put clothes away in cupboards and have a minimum of furniture.

Colour Therapy

History
The ancient Egyptian and Greeks used colour in their healing, as well as gemstones and crystals. In china people were wrapped in red silk and put out in the sun to cure chickenpox and Tibetan teaching recognize the power of colour in meditation and healing. The first scientific report was published in 1810 by Goeth called the theory of colour. Colour is now recognized and used widely; in shops, bars, hospitals and the workplace to evoke; mood, healing, relaxation and stimulation.

Theory
Colour plays a major part in all our lives, surrounding us and affecting everyone differently. Experts believe colour can alter our moods, emotions, health and well-being; various colours create a different atmosphere. Different people prefer to wear and surround themselves with particular colours: red may suit one person, yet be loathed by someone else. Colour can tell us a lot about whom we are, how we feel and what we want to achieve. The therapist will use colour to address various problems that an individual may have, from stress to insomnia, skin disorders, digestion problems and even emotional uncertainties.

We are constantly surrounded by colour in nature and our everyday environments, which most people take for granted. Those who work with colour, however, such as artists, designers and colour therapists, become acutely sensitive to its physical and psychological effects.

Other Information
The following colours can be useful for insomnia:

• Blue is a useful colour with which to treat tension, fear palpitations and insomnia it will reduce inflammation, and is used for laryngitis, sore throat, tonsillitis and goitres. It is also useful for shock, and headaches. When blue is administered with its complementary colour orange, it brings about a state of peaceful joy or hopeful peace. This makes it an excellent colour to use with meditation and in places of healing.

• Amethyst is reputed to help in headaches and cases of insomnia brought on by stress and tension, it is soothing to those suffering from sorrow and psychological ailments, bringing comfort and relief. The colour Indigo comprises blue and violet and is the dominant colour of the brow chakra. It works with the pituitary gland that controls the hormone balances in the body and encompasses the organs of sight and hearing combining both the blue and violet rays, it speaks of deep devotion, and love. Use blue and orange or indigo and gold or amethyst to help cure insomnia, use the crystals, decoration in you're bedroom and pictures and accessories in you home.

Crystals and Gemstones

History
The history of crystal therapy dates back into antiquity where certain gemstones represent different aspects of life and luck. Different gems have always represented different moods and aspects of our lives.

Theory
Connected to colour therapy is crystal and gem healing; the belief that crystals, precious and semi-precious gems have healing properties has a long history. The emerald was credited with the power to ward off epilepsy, cure dysentery and aid weak eyesight. Crystals and gems have long been used as symbols of power because they contain an earth

energy, which responds with the energies within the body to bring about healing.

Treatment
Crystals can be placed on corresponding parts of the body to help balance the controlling systems that manifest disease.

Crystals are often used with other therapies, like colour, reflexology and spiritual healing. Crystals are often used in Reiki healing. Crystal therapists maintain that crystals can help relieve spiritual, mental and physical ailments.

Relevance to insomnia
Some crystals are very calming and the correct use can help you to relax and to sleep.

Other information
The following colours of crystals and gems can help insomnia:

• All violet stones like amethyst and fluorite, violet stones are said to be spiritual and correspond with the highest elements in nature. The darker stones are associated with sorrow, deep purple signifies high spiritual attainment, and pale lilac indicates cosmic consciousness and a love for humanity, bluish purple stands for transcendental idealism. For healing, violet is said to be an aid for insomnia or for any ailment that relates to mental disorders.

• Blue stones like sapphire, lapis lazuli; blue is the symbol of inspiration, devotion, and infinity. It produces a calm peaceful radiation, which has sleep inducing qualities. For healing, blue carries great curative power in regard to any disease or blockage in the throat, it is cooling, sedative, astringent and healing. The deep dark blues indicate a power of tremendous intensity while the light blue indicates high ethical inspiration.

• Green stone like emerald, and, malachite, are all said to be beneficial for insomnia. Green is the symbol of harmony, sympathy, health, and abundance, of nature in general. Green reaches towards the horizon and blue reaches upwards. For healing green is important to the nervous system. It has a strong influence on the heart and will help heart problems, blood pressure, and restoring tired nerves.

Keep a crystal under the pillow or near the bed to counter nightmares and help you sleep, buy a chakra set of stones and keep them in a bag under your pillow. Crystals can enhance many different ambiences and you can choose them according to the mood you wish to create. There are certain stones that may aid restful sleep, for example, to help understand your dreams, keep a double terminated rock crystal close by while you sleep. To promote deep healing sleep, try putting a tumble polished piece of hematite under your pillow. To help oppose nightmares, place a large, smooth piece of moss agate or tektite by the bed where you can reach out and touch it. Its solid, reassuring feel will help to calm you if your sleep is a broken. When insomnia is a wearisome problem, try gazing into a small sphere of tumbled-shape of green aventurine. Its soft gentle hues and sparkling spangles of mica can help lull you to sleep.

The crystal rose quartz is associated with the heart chakra and can help with panic attacks and palpitations, wear a rose quartz pendent or buy a polished stone or heart shaped rose quartz crystal to place over your heart when you have an attack.

During an attack of palpitations put the crystal on your heart and place one hand lightly on top of it, breath deeply, breath into and feel the power of your heart. It can also help to repeat an affirmation to yourself, such as 'I am strong, I can overcome, and I can rest now.'

Insomnia Colour Exercise

Breathing in colour is a wonderful way of working with insomnia.

Try the following exercise. Firstly, make sure that your body is comfortable and warm. Mentally go over your body releasing any tension (as in the relaxation techniques in chapter 15). After you have done this, visualize a beautiful deep blue, and on each inhalation, take this colour into your body. Feel it encompassing every muscle, organ and cell. If it helps, you can imagine your body to be a very special container, which you are slowly filling with blue light. Continue to do this until you drift into sleep. Do not be disappointed and give up if your initial attempts fail. All that is needed is patient practice. You might also try sleeping in a blue nightdress or pyjamas between blue sheets. Also you may find that having a low wattage blue light burning during the night can also help restful sleep. I often burn a night-light or burner with a very low dose of essential oil in my bedroom, particularly if I am upset of restless and this helps me.

Yin and Yang

In considering the harmonious flow of Chi, the Chinese draw on the concepts of yin and yang. Chi energy is both yin and yang. Yin is often depicted as female energy, where male energy is yang. Heaven is seen as male and the earth as female.

What is between has to develop a balance between male and female so that harmony and balance can follow. As well as being male, yang energy is seen as active, light and expansive, where yin energy is regarded as passive, dark and receptive. Too much 'male' energy is harmful, just as too much 'female' energy is.

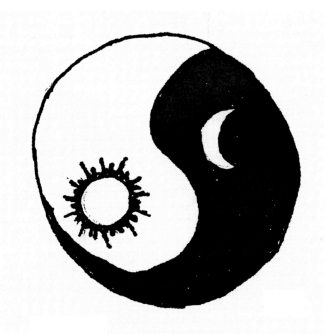

Harmony is achieved when yin and yang energy are in balance, Yin and Yang are not seen as being in conflict, they depend on each other. Deficiencies of the yin and the blood of the heart can bring on insomnia, memory loss irregular or racing heartbeat, excessive dreaming, and irrational behavior. Reiki can be very beneficial in balancing Yin and Yang energies

It is vitally important therefore that the flow of Chi is harmonious; this is not seen as a luxury but a necessity for happy, healthy and harmonious lives. If Chi is already flowing harmoniously, it can often be enhanced to further encourage growth, well-being, and good fortune by practising Feng Shui.

A relaxed body is essential for a sound sleep; Eastern sciences (such as Yoga) have known for thousands of years that the mind and body are connected and that they must be at one with each other. So it the mind is not relaxed, the body is not relaxed, and the body has to be relaxed for the mind to be relaxed, it's a package deal. Toe Wiggling is a technique that can help this process.

Toe Wiggling Exercise

Lie on your back and wiggle you toes up and down 12 times, wiggling the toes of both feet at the same time. This will relax your entire body, inside and out. How it works is connected to reflexology, and the belief that your feet are a kind of master control panel for the rest of your body. Meridians in the body channel energy from your feet and your hand to every organ in your body. When you wiggle your toes (or fingers) you are stimulating and thus relaxing your entire body, and energizing it at the same time. You can enhance the feeling by imagining that you are lying on a tropical beach and wiggling your toes in the hot sand or the warm waves are lapping over them.

Let your imagination run wild, as long as you feel warm, safe and secure you will feel relaxed and sleepy in no time.

Chapter 21

Natural Remedies

Homeopathy

History
In the eighteenth century Dr Samuel Hahnemann, a great German physician, was appalled by the medical practices of the day. He sought a method of healing which would be safe, gentle and successful. He believed that human beings have a capacity for healing themselves and that the symptoms of disease reflect the individuals struggle to overcome illness. Over a long period Hahnemann and his assistants took small doses of various substances, and carefully noted the symptoms they produced, he found that a minuscule amount of a substance that caused a symptom could also cure it.

Theory
Homeopathy is based on the premise that 'like cures like'. This means that if a substance produces symptoms (onions cause burning eyes) in a healthy person, it will cure those same symptoms in an unhealthy person (e.g. hay fever). Homeopathic remedies are made from various plants, minerals, metal, animal products and human products. Homeopathic philosophy is based on the belief that symptoms are signs of the body's effort to throw off disease; thus by repressing those symptoms one is impeding the healing process of the body.

One must treat the whole person not the symptoms taking into account the temperament of the person and his/her responses to medications on an individual bases.

Treatment
Your homoeopath will seek to strengthen the body's own ability to heal itself, believing the body can cope with most chronic and acute illnesses. Chosen correctly, a remedy will often stimulate a healing crisis, the temporary aggravation of symptoms. This is a good sign, as long as the reaction is not too severe. Homeopathy can help many ailments; allergies, respiratory problems, intestinal problems, and stress related diseases that often cause insomnia. All remedies have been diluted, which makes them safe to take. Homeopathic remedies should always be used one at a time and never together, it is preferable to consult a trained homoeopath. Care must be taken if using prescribed medicines, or undergoing other therapies like aromatherapy. Always inform your medical practitioner of use of homeopathic remedies.

Homeopathic remedies are available from many pharmacies and health shops, and some specialist suppliers.

Relevance to insomnia
Homeopathy can be very relevant to insomnia by treating the insomnia itself or by treating the underlying causes such as; stress, hay fever, night sweats ect.

Warning
Some homeopathic remedies should not be taken with other traditional medications, consult your doctor. Homeopathy does not mix well with aromatherapy. And you should only take one remedy at a time unless otherwise instructed by your therapist.

Other Information
Homeopathic remedies to try for insomnia:

• Aconite, use this for acute insomnia caused by shock or grief, if anxious and restless, travel sickness, bereavement, anxiety restlessness, fear and suffering from nightmares, with much twisting and turning in bed unable to get comfortable. If a warm room makes the condition worse, too many bedclothes, cold winds or cigarette smoke and made better by the open air and lighter bedclothes.

• Arsenicum Album, use for restlessness, anxiety and fear, cramps in calves, aversion to the smell of food, waking in early hours of morning with an over active mind. If condition is made worse by cold and wet weather, after eating cold ice cream or cold drinks and if made better by keeping warm.

• Arnica, use after an injury, for bruises and sprains or exercise, for over tiredness, for sensitivity to pain, gout, rheumatism, fear of being touched, unable to get comfortable and restlessness in bed. If condition is made worse by being touched, from motion and damp cold conditions and is made better from lying down with head low.

• Belladonna, use for swollen joints, restless night syndrome, Leg jerks in sleep, nightmares, earache, and headache, air sickness, and general disturbed sleep. If condition is made worse by lying down, from noise and touch and at night and is made better by keeping warm and sitting erect.

• Calc. Carb, use with sweating of the head during sleep, overweight, excessive appetite, constipation, itching skin and cracked hands in winter, period and premenstrual tension, menopause and night sweat that can disturb sleep. If condition is made worse when cold, damp, from standing too long or at night and if made better when warm or in dry weather.

• Ignatia, use when there is frequent yawning and watery eyes but you can't get to sleep, limbs become restless or hot and must be placed outside bedclothes, for emotional individuals, bereavement, grief, and headaches. If condition is made worse by cold air, strong odours tobacco smoke, coffee and alcohol and it is made better by warmth and fresh air.

• Kali-phos, use with nervous tension that builds up in the day and prevents sleep, mental tiredness from overwork, indigestion, headache, night terrors and humming in the ears following mental effort. If the condition is made worse by noise, excitement, worry and mental and physical exertion and if made better during gentle movement, from warmth and after nourishment.

• Pulsatilla, use for hay fever, change of life, menstrual pain, cystitis, tinnitus, sensitive people with fear of rebuke and rejection, if worry or early waking is stopping you sleep and dislike of extremes of weather. If made worse by heat, eating rich food and eating late in the evening, and sudden chilling when hot and if made better by open air, cold food and drink.

• Sepia, use for sadness and fear of being alone, mourning, difficulty falling asleep and waking unrefreshed, change of life, hot sweats and especially women who are easily depressed. If condition is made worse by afternoon and evening cold, before thunder, and from tobacco smoke and if made better by warmth.

• Sulphur, use for digestive problems, itching skin, acne, tendency to sweat, body odour, tinnitus, and interrupted sleep. If condition is made worse by cold and damp at the coast and made better by warm fresh air.

Naturopathy

History

Naturopathy, or naturopathic medicine, is a combination of a wide variety of natural therapeutics and healing techniques. A mixture of traditional folk wisdom and modern science passed down from to the Egyptians to the Greeks. Hippocrates believed in working in harmony with the natural lows that govern homeostasis, the body's drive to return to a state of equilibrium in health. The term naturopathy was coned by a nineteenth century German homeopath, John H. Scheel, to indicate health promotion of the whole person by natural means. Naturopathic medicine is the West's version of the many other nature-based and holistic medical systems in the world, like Ayurveda, traditional Chinese Medicine, and other natural health systems. Naturopathic Medicine is now practiced all over the world.

Theory

Most natural therapists believe that the body is losing its natural instincts to exercise, sleep naturally, eat, drink and combat stress causes illness. Naturopaths recommend a return to a more natural life-style in order to re-establish the connection between body and mind and the healing power of nature, this is achieved by making the individual more resilient and the immune system stronger. The philosophy is based on the fact that the body has its own healing process and will return to health and this process can be helped with the correct guidance provided by naturopathy.

Treatment

The first session will require the therapist taking a detailed consultation of the patient's history and making a clinical diagnosis. The naturopathic physician may order lab tests, and even an X ray or ultrasound, if necessary. Many will perform an osteopathic diagnosis, checking for misaligned structure of posture, the other main concern will be the patients diet and one may be asked to fill out a three of five-day food diary for analysis. The treatment program can consist of diet advice, home remedies, herbal teas, hot baths, massages, colonics and a mixture of other therapies such as acupuncture.

Relevance to insomnia
Naturopathic medicine can be very helpful for insomnia sufferers as it helps to balance the body and the mind, it is most often some imbalance in these areas that is causing the sleep problems.

Warning
Naturopathic medicine requires the patient to change their way of life there may be some detrimental emotional and physical reactions to treatment before a more balanced state of mind and body it achieved.

Herbalism

History
Herbal medicine differs from many other systems of alternative medicine because; it does not belong to any one culture, nor was it the inspiration of any one person. Herbs have been used for healing in nearly every known culture in the world for centuries. Herbalism is a vital part of Chinese medicine and Ayurvedic medicines. Therefore a vast amount of information has been acquired about which herbs help which organs and functions of the body. Herbs can now be prescribed accurately to heal sickness; herbs have also been used as a source of drugs in scientific medicine. Modern medicine traces its roots back to the Greek philosopher Hippocrates, who wrote about plant remedies. Many parts of the world still rely on local vegetation as their medicine chests. Scientists explore the curative powers of native plants, hoping to distil their active ingredients into modern drugs.

Theory
Herbal medicines are said to work biochemically, triggering neurochemical responses in the body. Taken in moderate doses for long enough, these biochemical responses become automatic, even after one stops taking the herbs.

Herbalism is very suitable for those who are prepared to take the remedies regularly and who do not expect instant results.

Treatment
Herbal remedies often take time to prepare and are particularly appropriate for people who enjoy the ceremony of preparing their evening infusion and have the time to do so. Herbal remedies offer a safe and non-addictive alternative to sleeping pills.

Relevance to insomnia
A helpful aid for insomnia and for stress and depression related conditions. Herb teas can be particularly helpful see details below.

Warning
Herbs can be slow acting, gentle medicinals, ideal for treating ailments like allergies but always consult a qualified practitioner and inform your doctor of remedies taken. Over the counter teas are quite safe.

Other information
Try drinking a camomile, catnip or lime flower tea, or an infusion of passionflower, valerian, or hops with 1/2 part licorice. Herb teas are available at all good health shops or from an herbalist and should be drank when stressed and before going to bed. You could also try relaxing in an herbal bath a Lime Blossom, lavender baths. Make a muslin bag and fill it full of herbs and tie the bag on to the hot tap so that the hot water runs through it. The Valerian bath is also excellent to promote restful sleep. Pour a litre of boiling water onto one

or two handfuls of the dried root of Valerian, leave it to stand for half an hour, then strain the liquid and add it to the hot bath, which should be taken just before going to bed. The bath may be a whole bath, a foot or hand bath. One of valerians active components is 'valepotriates', which has similar components to tranquilizers like diazepam (Valium), but without the side effects.

Another effective sleep aid is to drink two teaspoons of cider vinegar and one of honey, mixed into a cup of hot water. In may be that the calcium and other trace elements in this mixture have a soothing effect on the nervous system and so induce sleep.

Herbs to try for insomnia:

• California Poppy, gentle and non-addictive, a good alternative to the Opium Poppy, hypnotic, tranquillizer and anodyne (pain relieving) safe for children. Use as a tea at night to promote restful sleep.

• Camomile Roman, calming, soothing, and tonic. Use as tea at night, in baths, as an essential oil in massage oils, in burners and you can also put two drops on your pillow at night to calm you and aid sleep. Safe for children, but avoid internal use during pregnancy.

• Cowslip, sedative and antispasmodic, excellent for stress related problems, use as a tea, up to three times a day.

• Ginkgo Biloba, helps oxygen and nutrients reach the brain due to narrowing arteries and diminishing circulation. Good for circulation problems like cold feet and hands, headaches and migraine, senility, concentration, tinnitus and vertigo, and can be taken in capsule form.

• Hops, sedative, hypnotic and anodyne, calms excess excitability. Use as tea at night, hop pillows are available and aid sleep. High consumption is not advisable for men as hops contain the female hormone oestrogen and that is why men who drink a lot of beer get saggy chests and big tummies, and can start to grow breasts, they may also lose their sex drive.

• Jatamansi (Indian Valerian root) is superior to western Valerian because is promotes awareness, relaxation and strengthens the mind. Western Valerian dulls the mind after long-term use. Jatamamsi is one of the best herb for nervous disorders, insomnia, sleeplessness, vertigo, fainting and hysteria. It can be eaten directly from the jar, made into a tea 4 hours before bedtime.

• Passionflower, Sedataive, hypnotica and anodyne, calms the nervous system and promotes sleep. Avoid high doses in pregnancy.

• Saint Johns Wort, Sedative, restorative tonic for the nervous system, ideal for depression and aiding restful sleep, good for intestinal problems and diarrhoea, can also help children suffering from incontinence, it can be taken as a infusion or in tablet form.

• Valerian root, very potent tranquillizer, antispasmodic and mild anodyne. Take as an infusion or tea, also available in tablet form. Don't take for prolonged periods, may lead to over-exitedness.

• Wild Lettuce, Sedative, once known as the poor man's opium, take as an infusion or tincture before going to bed, the fresh leaves can also be eaten in salads. Excess can lead to insomnia and increased sexual activity, lower doses can cause sleepiness, so avoid if driving.

Many of these herbs, and some others, can be taken as a tea/infusion, tinctures in which herbal essences are infused in alcohol, and in tablet/capsule or extract form. They are all good for helping to overcome insomnia, especially when stress and depression are a contributing factor.

Herbs can be slow acting, gentle medicinal, and an alternative or complementary treatments for chronic conditions like allergies and insomnia. It is best not to rely on one herb on any regular basis, but to rotate among several. There are many good books available that will give you the medicinal and culinary uses of herbs, or consult a qualified herbalist for the medical effects.

Wheat pillows and herb pillows are also very good at promoting restful sleep, you can buy them ready made or make your own. Make a simple fabric pocket and fill it with wheat and herbs and then stitch up the sides, and then place it under your own pillow.

• For insomnia use hops, wild oregano, dill, sweet marjoram and lavender.

• To stimulate dreams use the following; peaceful dreams; sage, balsam, or safras; for more vivid dreams use mugwort, mint, lavender or lemon balm;
for dreams of love and romance use rose, yarrow, or basil.

• To remember your dreams use rosemary, lavender, catnip or bay.

• To banish nightmares use rosemary, valerian, or lemon balm.

• To help with headaches use marjoram, dried roses, lavender or bay.

• For despair or heartache use roses, dill, basil, or coriander.

Wheat pillows and wheat and herb pillows can be heated in the microwave for use with aches, pains and headaches, and they make an ideal alternative to a hot water bottle, they are also very safe for children. They can also be cooled in the fridge for sprains and swollen limbs.

Bach Flower Remedies

History
Bach flower remedies are a simple, natural and effective system of medicine. Dr Edward Bach developed them in the 1930's, a noted doctor, Homoeopath, bacteriologist and immunologist, who believed that a healthy mind is the key to recovery from ill health. Together the 38 remedies help you manage your emotions, working gently to restore balance and emotional well-being.

Theory
Bach supposed that emotions such as guilt, fear, or doubt create personality obsessions, which would eventually lead to physical consequences, stress, pain and sickness. Bach's most famous remedy is a combination of five flowers, called Rescue Remedy, available at any health shop, and a good standby for stressful situations. Used in emergency situations or for trauma, Rescue Remedy helps reduce the effect of trauma and marshal the body's own healing powers.

Treatment
A Bach flower practitioner will take a detailed consultation and then prescribe a combination of essences for you to take. For children and babies one needs to consider the behaviour and temperament, a qualified therapist will take all aspects of a persons life and personality into account when choosing the correct essences for a patient.

Many ready made remedies can now be purchased in health shops and they are very effective. A standard dose is 6-7 drops under the tongue. For specific ailments it is better to find a Bach Flower practitioner to tailor make combinations for your needs.

Bach Flower remedies are quite safe to use for children and even animals respond well to them, when a child is ill, or showing behavioural difficulties Bach flower remedies can be very effective

Relevance to insomnia
Bach flower essences can be very helpful for insomnia sufferers either by treating the insomnia itself or by addressing the contributory factors such be it stress, hay fever or night sweats.

Other Information
Flower remedies to try for insomnia:

• Aspen, use in cases of fear, panic attacks, foreboding or dread, night sweats, sleepwalking and sleep talking.

• Black-eyed Susan, use for impatience, those unable to unwind, preoccupied and unable to suppress painful old memories and emotions.

• Cherry Plum, use in periods of anxiety or depression and for those in a desperate frame of mind, on the verge of a nervous breakdown, suicide or madness or when one twists and turns in bed and can't rest.

• Dill, use for jet lag, stressful situations or for the over excited, safe and suitable for children.

• Morning Glory, use for those with eccentric sleep habits, can't get up in the morning, or are recovering from addictions, sleeping pills, drugs or cigarettes.

• Rock Rose, use for fear and terror, ideal to use for bad dreams and nightmares, night terrors and sleeplessness conditions brought on by stress and accidents.

• Valerian, use for stress, those in pain and kept awake because they are uncomfortable, also for people recovering from illness or upset in their lives.

• Verbena, use for highly wired, hyperactive, and tense people who can't unwind, use only at bedtime.

• Vervain, use for people that are frustrated and tense, unable to unwind, people who push themselves too hard and can't relax, Vervain remedy help people to wind down so that they can relax and give themselves a chance to rest. Take only before bedtime.

• Walnut, use at times of change, new job, new home, or new environment, it helps cut old ties and start afresh, helpful at puberty, menopause, and after childbirth. use walnut for sensitive people who are easily disturbed by outside influences and lose sleep over worry.

• White Chestnut, use this remedy for the tormented, worried, and obsessed, those that can't stop fretting over something and are unable to concentrate. White Chestnut remedy helps to relieve the mental whirlpool and restore peace of mind.

• Ylang Ylang, use for jet lag and insomnia brought on by stress, change and emotional upheaval. Ylang Ylang is calming, soothing, relaxing and can be aphrodisiac.

Chapter 22

Nutrition and Nutritional Therapies

Food and Nutritional Therapy

History

In primitive times, obtaining and eating food consumed most of humanity's time and energy. Food and water are the basic substance of our life our fuel. Food is so basic to life that, along with herbs, it is our first medicine. In ancient civilizations it was the only medicine. The science of nutrition and nutrition therapies is well established today in all parts of the world. Metabolic researchers have been putting together a picture of proteins, carbohydrates, and fates, as well as vitamins and minerals, as essential to human life and health. The 1940's scientists had identified more that 40 nutrients contained in foods, including 13 vitamins. They also determined that we need minerals, such as calcium, iron and potassium; to regulate various body functions. Beyond general nourishment, food and diet have been used throughout history as effective tools in preventive and therapeutic medicines. Recently we have begun to recognize once again and to investigate the valuable role that nutrition can play in a comprehensive health programme. Nutrition therapies, such as Orthomolecular Medicine/psychiatry, are used to help treat diseases like schizophrenia.

236

Theory

Our eating patterns are very important because our digestive systems are partly controlled by our natural biological rhythms. These natural rhythms allow us to anticipate large meals by providing enzymes before the food arrives to aid digestion.

Treatment

A therapist of dietitian will ask you to fill in a weeklong food diary; they will also do a detailed consultation about your health and lifestyle. The therapist will then recommend a diet or specific food remedies that can include vitamin and mineral supplement.

Relevance to insomnia

Nutritional therapy can be a very valuable aid in getting a good nights sleep by eating the right foods and at the right times. Many doctors' surgeries now have a dietitian ask for a referral. Some foods are better eaten separately (see page 242 for information on food combining).

Warning

Some foods can cause allergies and it is never recommended to eat only one kind of food all the time, variation is best.

Other information

Eating a large heavy meal within three/four hours of bedtime will increase your metabolic rate and your body temperature at a time when they should be decreasing.

This makes it harder to get to sleep because your body will still be working hard to digest food. Although it is often the case that you feel sleepy after a meal during the day, this is because your body temperature is already high and the increased effort to digest food causes a move away from metabolism in your muscles, promoting inactivity and sleepiness. This is more effective if alcohol is also consumed, a large meal and an alcoholic drink at lunchtime will frequently make you feel drowsy in the afternoon.

While it is equally obvious that disturbed sleep may arise from a stuffed feeling following a heavy meal or eating late in the evening, as well as from hunger pangs, other factors in food play their part. We live in an over stimulated world, and this has spread to the food we eat and the drinks that we imbibe.

Insomnia often afflicts busy people who never have enough time to eat properly or correctly, they are sometimes extroverts who have trouble being able to switch off their minds, and their digestive system will also suffer from not stopping to relax over a meal. You may be unable to sleep for many reasons, perhaps you are over-tired, have worries and concerns or perhaps your digestive system is too full with food, or the wrong food.

Fasting

Fasting does not always interfere with sleep, and many people will find that they sleep better during and after a fast.

Fasting produces a fall in body temperature; a similar fall in body temperature is found in natural sleep. A period of fasting combined with sufficient rest and warmth may actually be conducive to sleep. Abstention from food frequently produces a sense of lightness, well being and freedom from tension.

These characteristics are an important development in the promotion of sound sleep.

Fasting would only be contra-indicated where a state of severe physical and mental exhaustion has been reached and where a condition of neurosis forbids the use of the fasting technique. For all others, however, fasting may be used safely as a means of cleansing the system of an acid imbalance and preparation for easier sleep.

To go through a fast of any length, except under medical supervision, would be unwise. The normal healthy person can, however, easily manage a three-day fast at home. To obtain the best results, the fast should be carried out over a period where one can rest. At such times, even if you do not sleep, the inclined positions favourable to sleep, and any extra rest which can be gained is an advantage, for it will encourage the relaxation, which is always conducive to sleep.

To commence the fast, take a dose of Epsom salts dissolved in a little warm water, together with a large tumbler of boiled water, allowed to cool, and add a piece of orange or lemon. Repeat this half an hour later and throughout the next three days at regular intervals.

There are many kinds of fasts and many books are available to help you choose the right one for you.

The Right Foods

Plenty of fresh fruit and salads, dried fruits, green and root vegetables, live yoghurt, brown rice, oats, wholemeal bread and flour, pulses and beans, fish and free-range chicken rather than red meats, also limit eggs and hard cheese. There are benefits associated with eating fish, particularly oily fish, a low-fat protein which is a rich source of essential fatty acids, which help maintain a healthy cardiovascular system and improve the condition of skin, hair and nails.

Root vegetables are said to be more sedative that leaf vegetables. Have your main protein meal midday and a lighter carbohydrate meal early evening, if you get hungry later in the evening have a banana, some dried fruit and nuts or a sweet biscuit or whole grain cracker with a milky drink or a herb tea one hour before going to bed, these foods contain tryptophan, which promotes sleep.

Foods to Avoid

Cut out or avoid sugar and refined foods, cut down on stimulants, tea, coffee, chocolate, and cola drinks. Drink lots of pure water at least 1 to 2 litres everyday, water and fresh fruit juices are vital to a healthy circulation. Try putting a jug of water with a slice of lemon in it in the fridge and every time you open the fridge door have a glass of water.

Now to some following this advice, there may seem good reason to feel depressed, but believe me after a few weeks, when you wake up in the morning refreshed and ready to face the world, you will feel very differently. My tip is to have a big bowl full of different fresh fruits, and a jar with different nuts and dried fruits in it. The thing is that you don't have to cut out all your favourite things, just don't make them a crutch to get through bad times, but a reward for the good times.

Sugar in all its forms (cakes, chocolate, sweets), refined carbohydrates (white flour and sugar), processed foods (full of E numbers and additives), high saturated fat foods (full fat cheese, fatty meat) these put a extra strain on your digestive system particularly if eaten in the evening.

Caffeine, (found not just in coffee, tea, colas, chocolate and many other soft drinks) avoid caffeine in the evening it will make you hyperactive.

Excess salt (raises blood pressure) we get all the salt we need naturally from our food, and only need extra in hot climates when we will sweat more that usual.

Avoid bacon, cheese, chocolate, eggplant, ham, potatoes, sugar, sausage, spinach, tomatoes, and wine close to bedtime. These foods contain tryramine, which increases the release of norepinephrine, a brain stimulant.

Avoid the foods that give you heartburn, especially within three hours of bedtime, and meals that are spicy, heavy, fatty, and greasy or protein rich in the evening.

When to eat

The old saying 'breakfast like a king, lunch like a lord and dine like a pauper', makes a lot of sense. Our digestive system works more slowly as the day goes on, and a heavy meal in the evening means that your body is working hard to digest food instead of concentrating on resting and going to sleep.

If you habitually sleep badly, a large breakfast is definitely the best idea, also for those among us that want to loose a bit of weight eating early in the day and tapering of towards the evening will help a great deal. Eat whole grain bread and cereals, yoghurt, fruit, and fresh juice to maintain energy levels through the morning. For lunches go for lots of carbohydrates and vegetables and only small amounts of proteins like fish, chicken, eggs meat and cheese. Proteins stimulate the production of dopa or dopamine, this chemical converts into adrenaline and will help your energy levels through the afternoon. For your evening meal eat lightly and not too late in the evening, again carbohydrates such as jacket potato, pasta or brown rice are good choices and combine them with eggs and dairy produce and a little meat or fish, to produce the sedative amino acid tryptophan. If you are vegetarian have some nuts or pulses like lentils and beans. If you suffer from low blood sugar you may need a light snack before bedtime, keep this to the minimum, a good choice can be a lettuce or banana sandwich, a small bowl of cereal (no sugar) or peanut butter on toast with a glass of milk. These foods will also help produce trytophan and induce sleep.

By re-balancing your system and feeding your body earlier in the day, and working in co-operation with you body clock you can go a long way towards combating insomnia. More insomnia is caused by over-eating than by semi-starvation, if, however anything is required during the night, a few grapes or a digestive biscuit could be kept in a handy position by the bedside along with a glass of water.

Any natural distaste for food should, within intelligent bounds, be recognized and obeyed, it is an instinct that could prevent many a wakeful night, and could be an indication of food allergies.

Try drinking a glass of water and then putting a pinch of salt on your tongue. My personal experience, and observation in others, has shown that one begins falling asleep within a few minutes. According to Dr F Batmanghelidj in his book *Your body's many cries for water*'this combination alters the rate of electrical discharge in the brain and induces sleep. Remember not to touch the palate with the salt because that may cause irritation. Try leaving a jug of cold water with a squeeze of lemon in it, in the fridge and every time you open the door have a small glass of water. You can also make up herbal teas and cool them in the fridge, this makes a delicious summer drink.

Food Combining

Stress can cause appetite problems, indigestion, stomach upsets and diarrhoea. It can produce headaches, muscle tension, clenched jaws and grinding teeth. Food combining which, in a nutshell, is a diet based on not mixing protein and starch in the same meal can help combat stress.

People's digestive systems work better for not having to work on too many different kinds of foods in one meal. A good rule of thumb is to eat fresh foods not processed foods, don't eat the same foods every day, but have plenty of variety and to keep to regular meal times every day. Foods are digested differently, i.e. protein and carbohydrate are better eaten separately to ease the digestion process.

There certainly have been great improvements for people with nervous tummies and Irritable Bowel Syndrome (IBS) and Diverticulosis from following a food combining diet.

Caffeine Intake Coffee, Tea, Soft Drinks

A common origin of insomnia, that many people fail to identify as a problem, is caffeine. Many people talk about having a cup of coffee to wake them up or to get them going, but few realize that caffeine, under some circumstances, can increase sleepiness.

A cup or two of coffee or tea may be okay, unless you're unusually sensitive to caffeine, but anything more than that should be eliminated. Overuse increases anxiety and interferes with the body's natural regulation process. Plan to cut down your caffeine intake, avoid caffeinated drinks at times of stress, don't get into a routine of drinking caffeine, coffee while studying for example, try one day a week without caffeine.

Don't be surprised if you have withdrawal symptoms when cutting down. Caffeine is an addictive substance and is also found in many soft drinks such as coke. It is not advisable to drink any caffeinated beverages after 6 pm and certainly not before going to bed.

Melatonin

Many people that have been able to restore normal sleeping patterns by with melatonin. Melatonin is a substance produced in the brain by the pineal gland; a pea-size structure nestled at the center of the brain, when it is stimulated by light entering the eye. Melatonin is the hormone that keeps our brains in balance with the rhythms of the day and of the seasons.

During the short days of winter, melatonin levels become so low in some people that a condition called Seasonal Affective Disorder (SAD) or Winter Blues develops. (see page..) this condition can be helped by melatonin supplementation and/or exposure to full-spectrum lighting. (see useful addresses appendix 1) As people get older the production of melatonin declines and middle aged adults secrete only half as much as children. Melatonin is not a drug, it is much safer than tranquillizers or sleeping pills, it is non-toxic, and is relatively cheap. Melatonin has shown to be sedative and to improve the quality and duration of sleep; it is also helpful for shift-workers, for jet lag and many stress related conditions.

Melatonin is also reputed to help keep at bay the signs of aging, by extending life and helping with memory loss, protecting cells from free radicals, boosting the immune system and preventing cancer. These hormones can be prescribed by your doctor or purchased from some health shops.

Serotonin

Serotonin is a neural transmitter, which calms the system. A basic source of serotonin is L-Tryptophan, an amino acid found in foods such as sweet biscuits and sweet crackers. Eat one of these sweet foods before bed and chew slowly. This will liberate the sugar to produce serotonin in your brain and relax your body. Reduce the amount of protein in your food and eat fewer milk and dairy products to lower your acid level. The combination of serotonin and a lower acid level will act as a powerful soporific.

Serotonin is now only available on prescription from a medical practitioner.

DHEA

Dehydroepisterone (DHEA) is a naturally occurring hormone that improves the quality of sleep. DHEA can be taken as a supplement, it is also credited with helping delay the aging process, deter cancer and help with diabetes and Parkinson's disease.

Supplements for Insomnia

• Multivitamin and multimineral one a day supplement

• Vitamin B6 100mg with zinc 10mg (vitamin B6 must be taken with zinc, which is needed to convert B6 into its active form)

• Calcium 600mg to 1,500mg and magnesium 400mg to 1,000mg daily (can be taken before going to bed)

• 2 x K-Tryptophan 1000mg (only if absolutely necessary, and not for any prolonged period of time).

• All the B vitamins are beneficial, get a multi B supplement

• Melatonin start with 1.5mg daily, taken 2 hours or less before bedtime. Higher does can be taken, build up gradually if needed, up to 5mg daily.

• Inositol 100mg daily at bedtime enhances REM sleep. (obtainable on prescription only)

PART FOUR

Chapter 23

There are a thousand ways of pursuing sleep when it is evasive. Many of them command a great deal of merit and are applicable to many cases of insomnia. Other methods are satisfactory only to a limited number, and much of the advice that is given on the subject is helpful only to the individual who gives it. Courting sleep is just as much a personal affair as selecting the winning number in the lottery.

I truly believe that there are few sleep problems that cannot be overcome with time, patience and self-help. When you have tried some of the recommendations in this book, you will I hope have found the right answers for you personally. There is nothing wrong in any method, no matter how trivial or serious it may appear, if it serves the purpose of bringing about relaxing sleep.

If you still feel that after reading this book, there are serious insomnia questions for yourself or for someone you care for, if your sleep has been disturbed for more than a month and interferes with the way you feel or function during the day, you may well be advised to see your doctor, healthcare provider, or ask for a referral to a sleep disorders specialist, sleep clinic, for counselling or therapy. Your medical history, a physical examination, and laboratory tests, such as hormone function testing, may help identify certain causes.

246

Your bed partner and other household members may have useful information about your sleep, such as whether you snore loudly or sleep restlessly. Your doctor or sleep therapist will also need to know whether insomnia makes you sleepy or depressed or if it affects your life in any other ways. They will also need to know your work routine and activity levels, what exercise you take and what you do to relax.

Sometimes insomnia can be lessened through education and information; some people naturally sleep less than others, and merely need to abandon the misconceived belief that every body needs eight-hours of sleep every night. In cases of trauma, night terrors, behavioural problems and depression, counselling can help where these conditions are the contributory factors to insomnia and poor sleep. In other cases, medication or evaluation at a sleep disorder center or via a therapist may be prescribed. As part of the evaluation with any therapist or at a sleep disorder center the patient may be asked to keep a sleep diary showing sleeping and waking patterns for a week or two, this may help highlight specific areas of concern.

Choosing a Professional Therapist

Many of the remedies and exercises is this book are safe and easy to use at home, but not all remedies are effective for everyone and not all therapies suit everybody. Some people are more attracted to hands on therapies like massage and reflexology; others would prefer an herbal or homeopathic antidote, exercise or meditation. Many of the natural therapies are safe to use together, but always seek advice if you are in any way uncertain.

Your best recourse is to choose a therapist or therapists who you feel can combine their knowledge and your intuition.

When looking for a therapist, choose carefully make sure that they have the correct qualifications and that they are insured to practice their trade. It is advisable to contact the appropriate organization and ask for a list of credited practitioners.

You can also ask your doctor for a referral, your GP may not be very helpful, but don't be put off, ask around you may be able get a recommendation from a friend or colleague.

I have listed many useful addresses of professional organizations and registering bodies to help you find a qualified practitioner in each of the different therapies and treatments. It you are outside the UK, look in the phone book under the name of the treatment or therapy. In the USA you can contact the American Sleep Disorders Association who publish some very informative leaflets and have information on different therapies.

The most important factor in choosing health professionals is the match between their skills and your problem or goals. Being clear about what you need and want helps narrow the choices. It gives you clear-cut questions to ask the practitioner during the initial phase of the search. You should find out in advance the cost, and duration of treatments and if you are not sure ask exactly what is involved. The therapist should always take a detailed consultation, history of your health and other pertinent factors relating to your condition. Be open with them and don't hold back on aspects of your life that may be very relevant to your problem, i.e. personal worries about the family, your job or health. You must feel as ease with your therapist and trust them; they in turn must keep your personal details confidential.

If you don't feel as ease with your therapist, and visa versa, you will not achieve much, then you must change to someone you can relate to. If the experience was upsetting or unsatisfactory in any way, it is up to you whether you need to communicate that to the relevant authority, personal style, or personality clash is one thing, incompetence is another?

Getting a Good Night's Sleep Checklist

A routine will help to condition you to go to sleep, undressing, washing, cleaning your teeth, and any other particular personal observance you may have adopt a relaxing but not restricting ritual before going to bed:

General Tips and Environmental Factors

• Set an alarm clock and get out of bed at the same time every morning, try also to go to bed around the same time each night, this makes it much more likely that you will develop a regular time to get sleepy. Once normal sleep patterns are re-established, many people find that they have no need for an alarm clock.

• Don't lie in even at weekends, no matter how late you went to bed the night before.

• Try not to take your troubles to bed with you, stress keeps you awake, brooding on your problems makes them seem worse, and, if you're tired in the morning, less able to deal with them.

• If you have forgotten to do something, get up and write yourself a note, leave it somewhere prominent like on the kettle, to remind you to do it in the morning, then forget about it.

• If you are going to have an argument or a deep discussion with someone try not to do it just before you go to bed. Emotional stress and confrontation can lead to a disturbed night as you mull over what was said or what you could have said.

• Regular exercise during the day helps you to sleep, but it is not advisable to do any too energetic exercise within 3 hours of going to bed.

• Try learning some relaxation techniques and breathing exercises, these can help relieve stress, relax the mind and ease tense muscles.

• Make sure that the bedroom isn't too hot, or too cold; make sure the temperature is right for you, both in the room and in the bed.

• Make sure the room is properly ventilated but be beware of drafts from open windows.

• Chose a bedroom décor that is restful and relaxing to you, make your bedroom and your bed as comfortable as possible, sleep on a durable mattress, with adequate bedclothes.

• Consider the use of relaxing aromas in an Aroma-therapy fragrancer or safe burner/night light before bedtime.

• Try to limit noise and light, thick curtains, blinds and good double-glazing can help, consider earplugs to cut down on noise. Use thick lined curtains or blinds to cut down on light from the street.

• Check your medication, some common medication can cause insomnia.

• Don't take naps even if you're tired at a certain point in the day try to keep active or exercise at this time instead.

• If you are a shift worker try to establish a routine before bedtime, whatever the time of day. Eat your main meal before going on your shift and do not have a heavy meal before going to bed.

• Try different natural mineral and vitamin supplement supplement, find what's right for you, and alternate them, don't keep to the same thing for long periods.

Before Bed Time:

• Eat a light meal in the early evening or a very light snack no later that one-hour before bedtime. Eat a healthy, well balanced diet, having the larger meals earlier in the day.

• Avoid alcohol at bedtime many an insomniac's believes that an alcoholic drink helps them sleep, in fact, alcohol often has the opposite effect.

• Avoid too much fluid before bedtime partly because it can cause visits to the bathroom during the night.

• Avoid stimulants such as alcohol, nicotine and caffeine for a couple of hours before bed and remember that tea, coffee, cocoa, cola and some medications contain caffeine. Many people do find a cup of hot chocolate or horlicks beneficial to sleeping before going to bed.

• Take the dog, or yourself, for a gentle walk about hour before you go to bed

• Have a warm relaxing bath; keep the temperature slightly warmer than your own, body not too hot. Don't stay in the bath more than 20 minutes, and add some aromatherapy oils or a favourite bubble bath if is to your taste.

• Try hot milk, milky drinks, not tea of coffee, do help some people sleep. Milk helps because it contains tryptophan an amino acid that is a component of serotonin, part of the sleep hormone melatonin.

• Get your partner or a friend to give you a massage, or do some self-massage to your feet using some aromatic essential oils.

• Don't watch TV in bed, don't read anything too serious in bed, and don't take your work to bed with you. Use the bed for sleep and sex only.

• Listen to the radio, to music, relaxation tape, or read (avoiding highly emotion or work related topics)

• Half an hour at least before you go to bed prepare a list of thoughts, ideas, things to remember for the morning, get them out of your head and on to a piece of paper. Leave the list in another room or shut it away in a drawer

• Try yoghurt, a glass of milk or an herbal tea before bedtime.

• If you suffer from low blood sugar have a sweet biscuit before retiring.

• Listen to some gentle music, do a relaxation routine or sit and read for a while, sex is also a good relaxant.

Avoid the Following:

- Sleeping in the evening, for example in front of the television

- Taking cat-naps during the day or sleeping-in in the morning the attempt to catch upon lost sleep

- Carrying out over stimulating intellectual tasks just before bedtime.

- Carrying out work tasks in the bedroom particularly in bed

- Having electrical machinery, computers in the bedroom

- Watching exciting or frightening television or video programs before bedtime.

Some Tips for when you are in Bed:

- If you still can't sleep, don't lie there worrying about it, get up and do something, read or have a cold or milky drink, then go back to bed when you do feel tired.

- If you're lying in bed and can't stop your mind from racing, think of a short word like 'petal' and try repeating it over and over in your mind to block out any other thoughts. You can also try counting backwards from ten over and over again (10 9 8 7 6 5 4 3 2 1), this numbs the brain into turning off, and helps block out other thoughts that may be disturbing your rest.

- Do one of the relaxation or visualization exercises as outlines in chapter 15.

Conditioned Insomnia

Very few cases of insomnia are purely habitual; insomnia often starts with a short-term crisis or emotional upset, when the sufferer's routine, the bedroom and even the bed, become associated with unhappiness and sleeplessness. People whose insomnia is conditioned in this way often sleep well in strange beds when they go away. If this is the case change something, the room you sleep in, the decoration, the bed, the position of the bed, you may well find that this will help. Much conditioned insomnia starts in childhood; people who were sent to bed when they were small for being naughty may subconsciously associate bed and bedtime with anger and punishment. Some children are sent to bed for adult convenience long before they are really sleepy, they may then lie awake feeling bored and frustrated.

The negative feelings children get when they hear family rows, or when a child is sent to bed to get them out of the way, can make the bedroom become associated not with sleep but with sorrow and feeling alone.

You have to learn to associate the bedroom with sleep, don't have computers, television's, multigyms, don't study, or do active things in your bed room if possible.

If you have space restrictions and have to share your bedroom space with an office, for example, make sure that the two activities are well separated, by decoration, space or by a screen if possible.

Where possible use your bedroom for sex and sleep only, don't watch television, listen to the radio, read anything too stimulating, work, smoke or eat in bed, making love is permitted and in fact quite beneficial to sound sleep.

If after going to bed you don't fall asleep within 15/20 minutes, get up and do something else in another room. Don't go back to bed until you feel tired and ready to fall asleep. The same applies if you wake up in the middle of the night and can't get back to sleep, get up, make yourself a drink, read a book, or write a letter until you feel sleepy again. This method does not suit everybody, and can be a drag in the depth of winter, but it can be very successful.

Lying Awake

There are times when everybody has gone to bed and nothing has happened, but you just lie there wide-awake.

Don't just lie there frustrated, upset, or angry, which will make sleep even less likely, and will condition you to develop even worse sleep habits. In a single sweep we cannot deal with all the problems that have allowed insomnia to develop, probably over years but we can start to address the issues that are perpetuating it or making it worse.

Rather than there lie awake trying to get to sleep, get up and try again after a short period of activity, reading a book, having a cold drink, or doing some mundane chore of some kind. When you do get up keep yourself warm and comfortable, do something that is relaxing but involves no risk of your falling asleep before you can get back into bed. Avoid watching television and don't get into a habit of doing the same thing each time your sleep is disturbed and you get up in the night. When you feel sleepy go back to bed and try to sleep again, your aim is to associate being in bed with being sleepy, not with the frustration of not being able to get to sleep.

It can be helpful to hide your clock, or at least, turn the face so that you can't see the time during the night, clock watching can increase the frustration of lying in bed awake.

Don't be tempted to stay in bed longer in the morning after a restless night, get up at your normal time, be active during the day, and go to bed tired the next night. By lying in you are reinforcing an irregular sleep cycle and perpetuating the problem further. Be positive and tell yourself that tomorrow will be different, you will have a beautiful, restful and undisturbed sleep and wake refreshed and full of energy.

Even if you usually fall asleep easily, it is worth paying attention to simple practices that can improve the quality of your sleeping and waking hours, at some time in all our lives sooner of later almost everyone suffers from some kind of insomnia or sleep disturbance.

Breaking the 'habit' of Insomnia

The following strategy has proved to be most effective in breaking the habit of lying in bed and not going to sleep. It is probably a good idea to plan to use this strategy first when you expect a reasonably undemanding day the next day, and to warn other people in your household of your plan.

1. Move slowly through your helpful pre-bed routine, using ideas listed above.

2. When in bed use your favourite visualization or physical relaxation technique.

3. If you are not asleep 15 minutes after you have finished this GET OUT OF BED.

4. Leave the bedroom if at all possible and do some simple physical task. Clean your shoes, sew on a button, and polish a table. (If other people are in the house try to choose a quiet task!).

5. After 15 minutes return to bed, repeat the physical relaxation exercise, allow another 15 minutes for sleep to overcome you. Repeat if necessary all through the night.

6. NO NOT LIE IN BED WISHING TO SLEEP AND NOT SLEEPING.

If you use this strategy one night, even if you are up all night, you will certainly sleep the following night provided you don't allow yourself to catnap the following day. (and you will have clean shoes).

Sleep Diary and Dream Diary

Many people find it helpful to keep a diary, and record their sleep and dreams in it every morning. You will find that this can help you find out if there is a pattern to your insomnia and sleeplessness. For example, you may find that you have not slept well for the few days before a monthly period, or before an important meeting at work, or when you have eaten late in the evening or drunk alcohol or tea or coffee in the evening.

Finding out the triggers for your insomnia will help you to eliminate them or learn to deal with them. Recording your dreams will be very interesting, you can find out a lot about what is worrying you or what is going on in your life from your dreams, you will also find that once you start recording your dreams you will remember more of them, and it can make for some very interesting reading. Psychotherapists will tell us that our thoughts and imagination help shape the course of our lives, many of them advocate using the practice of creative imagery. Affirmation and visualization can really help, by imagining the way you want to feel until that is the way you do feel.

Sunday Night Insomnia

Many people have specific trouble sleeping on the night before the first working day of the week.

This can be part anxiety, part insomnia and part biological rhythms. And is similar to the effect of not sleeping before any meaningful day, big meeting or important event in your life. Anxiety about work is very common, and is exacerbated by weekend sleep schedules that are some times later and longer. You may have relaxed and slowed down at the weekend, and will find it difficult to get back into the working, rising early mode on return to work.

This can be a particular problem after any prolonged break from work such as a holiday, break due to illness or unemployment.

In this book I say that it is better to maintain a regular sleep cycle, going to bed and rising at the same time each day including weekends. Avoid, if possible, going to bed later than usual on Friday and Saturday nights. If you do stay up late on Saturday night, try to get up within an hour or so of your usual time on Sunday morning. Take some time on Sunday night, about half an hour, to review the coming working week, anticipate some of your concerns and plans, but then put these thoughts aside and go to bed knowing you are prepared for the coming working week.

Sleeping Away from Home

Some people find great difficulty sleeping away from home and not in their own bed. Others say that they can sleep like a baby when they are away on holiday or staying with friends. The important thing is to feel secure, take some personal effects away with you, to have something familiar to see when you go to bed, and see if that helps.

If you have more difficulty with sleep when you're away from your own home and your familiar surroundings and routine. You can help the problem by doing the following:

• Take your own pillow with you; use familiar, comfortable nightclothes and accessories so that you feel at home away from home.

• Take an emergency kit of the following items: ear plugs, eye shades, pain killers, antihistamines, essential oils and favourite complementary sleep remedies.

• In hotels and motels, request a quiet room, away from lifts, pool or bar.

• Check your room on arrival; adjust the temperature so that it will be right by bedtime. Ask the receptionist for extra blankets or pillows if your think you may need them, or a fan if the room is stuffy or too hot.

• If your room is not comfortable ask if you can move to another one.

• Speak to your doctor, therapist or health care provider before you leave home for extra medication or helpful suggestions when traveling.

• Take insect repellent and medications for tummy upsets, these are two sure fire aspects of a holiday that can keep you awake.

• When sleeping as a guest in someone else's house, follow the same precautions as before, but be sensitive to your hosts' routine before you go to bed, agree in advance times to be quiet and keep noise down and use bathing facilities and kitchen.

• Don't assume that because you are awake and ready for a cup of tea at 7 am in the morning that every one else in the house will be.

Sleepy when Driving

Falling asleep or sleepy while driving is extremely dangerous, it begins with a sleepy feeling, but often quickly progresses to head nodding and eyes closing and a struggle to control the vehicle correctly. One of its most dangerous aspects is the likelihood of 'microsleeps', which are short (5 to 8 second) lapses into sleep. The driver is usually unaware that these are happening, apart from having to struggle to remain alert. Up to 30/50 per cent of major accidents are caused by sleep at the wheel and alcohol brings out and intensifies and this sleepiness.

According to a recent report by the RAC Foundation:

• Insomnia is a silent killer, responsible for 350 deaths and up to 400 serious injuries on the UK's roads each year.

• Government statistic now confirms that driver fatigue or drowsiness may be a principal factor in 30 per cent of all road accidents.

• More than 60 per cent of driver's questioned admitted to having driven while sleepy and a startling eight per cent said that they had, at some time nodded off momentarily at the wheel.

• Thirty per cent also said that they felt more stressed, angry and more likely to confront other drivers when they were tired.

• The danger time for falling asleep at the wheel is between 4am and 6am when a motorist is 13 times as likely to have a sleep related accident as someone who is driving in the middle or the morning or early evening. Mid afternoon (2pm – 4pm) is also a danger period.

• Eleven per cent of all motorway accidents happen between 4am and 6am surprising, as traffic density is about a fifth of the average daily level during this time.

• The greatest incidence of sleep related accidents occurs when the driver has been awake for more than eighteen hours.

• Sleep apnoea, a medical condition that can result in "micro-sleeps" is a fairly common condition. Studies show that sufferers are seven times more likely to have a road accident than normal drivers.

Always think ahead, and plan long journeys or night driving schedules, arranging time for stops and breaks to eat or rest if and when needed. Wear comfortable shoes and clothes, play music or listen to the radio, and listen to something stimulating rather than mellifluous, to keep your attention and keep you awake. Talking books, or discussion type radio stations are best, also maintain a cool temperature in the car or have some fresh air, eating, drinking or chewing gum can help. There are differing opinions about talking on the phone, hands free, some say that it can be distracting while driving while others believe that it can keep you mind alert.

It can be beneficial to take a nap before you leave, eat a carbohydrate meal before setting out or plan to stop for a meal along the way and lastly and most importantly always drive considerately and safely so you do not get stressed and irritable during you journey.

We are all unique and therefore no one method can be guaranteed to suit everybody, try different things, and even when one works don't keep using the same method all the time but rotate different remedies. The ideas, therapies and remedies listed in this book can help you. Approach them with an open mind and practice each one for a sufficient length of time to allow yourself to make a proper assessment of their value to your by using your sleep diary. It is vital to have a positive attitude to your sleep and it is very important to develop healthy sleep habits that will take you through the rest of your life.

You too can re-discover the joy of natural and restful sleep.

Appendix 1

Useful addresses

For more information about Acupressure and Acupuncture send a large SAE to:
British Acupuncture council
Park House, 206/208 Latimer Road, London W10 6RE
(020 8964 0222)

Society of Auricular Acupuncture
Nurstead Lodge, Nurstead, Meophram, Kent DA13 9AD
(01474 813902)

The Acupressure Institute,
1533 Shattuck Avenue, Berkeley, California, 94709.

British Acupuncture council
Park House, 206/208 Latimer Road, London W10 6RE
0181 964 0222

For list of teachers for Alexander Technique send SAE to:
The Society of Teachers of the Alexander Technique.
20 London House, 266 Fulham Road, London SW10 9EL
0171 351 0828

Information for Allergy sufferers
British Society for Allergy, Environmental and Nutritional Medicine
P.O. Box 28, Totton, Southampton

For more information about Aromatherapy and a list of practitioners contact:

Aromatherapy Organizations Council
The Secretary, P.O Box 355, Croydon CR9 2QP
0181 251 7912

The Register of Qualified Aromatherapists
P.O. Box 3431, Danbury, Chelmsford, Essex CM3 4UA

International Federation of Aromatherapists
Stamford House, 2/4 Chiswick High Road, London W4 1TH
0181 742 2605

The Aromatherapy Trade Council
PO Box 52, Market Harborough, Leicester LE16 8ZX

Canadian Federation of Aromatherapy
P.O. Box 68571-1235, Williams Parkway East, Bramalea, Ontario
L6S6A1
(905) 457 6711

The National Association for Holistic Aromatherapy
P.O. Box 17622, Boulder, CO80308

For more information about Ayurvedic Physicians send a SAE to:

Association of Ayurvedic Physicians in the U.K.
1 Sybil Road, Rowley Fields, Leicester LE3 2EX
(0533) 892021

Maharisi Ayurveda Health Centers UK
Freepost WN5 5128, Skelmersdale, Lancashire WN8

Ayurvedic Living
PO Box 188, Exeter, Devon, EX4 5AY

Ayurvedic Company of Great Britain
50 Penywern Road, Earl's Court, London SW5 9SX

American Institute of Vedic Studies
P.O. Box 8357, Santa Fe, NM 87501
(505) 983 9385

For more information about Bach Flower remedies and practitioner list write to:
The Bach flower Centre
Mount Vernon, Sotwell, Wallingford, Oxfordshire, OX10 OPZ
(01491 834678)

For more information on the Bowen Method send a SAE to:
The Secretary
European College of Bowen Studies
38 Portway, Frome, Somerset, BA11 1QU
(01373 461873)

The Bowen Association
Powerpoint Business Centre, 122 High Street, Earlshilton, Leicester, LE9 7LQ
(01455 841800)

For more information about Chinese Herbal Medicine and practitioner list send a cheque for £2.50 and a SAE to:
Register of Chinese Herbal Medicine
PO Box 400, Middlesex HA9 9NZ
(020 7224 0883)

For more information about Chronic Fatigue Syndrome send a large SAE to:
Chronic Fatigue Syndrome Society
P.O. Box 230108, Portland, Oregon 97223
(503) 684 5261

For more information about chiropractic and a list of practitioners send a large SAE to:
British Association for Applied Chiropractic
The Old Post Office, Cherry Street, Stratton Audley, Nr Bicester, Oxen. OX6 9BA
(01869 277111)
(Send a cheque for £5.75)

The British Chiropractic Association
Blagrave House, 17 Blagrave Street, Reading, Berkshire RG1 1QB
(0118 950 5950)

(Send a cheque for £2.00)
McTimoney Chiropractic Association
21 High Street, Eynsham, Oxfordshire OX8 1HE
(01865 880974)

Scottish Chiropractic
16 Jenny Moores Road, St Bosells, Melrose, Roxburghshire
(01835 823645)

For more informatioin on Colonics and a list of practitioners send a SAE to:
Colonic International Association
16 Drummond Ride, Tring, Herts, SP23 5BE

For more information on Colour Therapy and practitioner list send and SAE to:
Aura Soma Colour Therapeutics
South Road, Tetford, Lincolnshire, NN9 6QB
(01507 533581)

The Colour Therapy Association
PO Box 16756, London SW20 8ZW
(020 8540 3540)

The International Association of Colour
P.O. Box 3, Potters Bar, Hertfordshire, ENG 3ET

The International Association for Colour Therapy
73 Elm Bank Gardens, Barnes, London SW13 0NX

International Association of Colour Therapy
P.O. Box 3 Potters Bar, London, EN6 3ET

For more information about Craniosacral Therapy and a practitioner list send a SAE to:
Craniosacral Therapy Association of the UK
27 Old Gloucester Street, London WCIN 3XX
(07000 784735)

The Upledger Institute UK
2 Marshall Place, Perth, PH2 8AH
(01738 444404)

For more information of Crystal Therapy and practitioner list send a large SAE to:

International Association of Crystal Therapy
PO Box 344, Manchester, M60 2EZ
(01405 769119)

International Federation of Crystal, Sound and Natural Therapy
35a Mayfield Road, Sanderstead, South Croydon, Surrey, CR2 OBJ
(020 8651 5247)

The School of Electro-crystal Therapy
117 Long Drive, South Ruislip, Middx HA4 OHL
(020 8841 1716)

Affiliation of Crystal Healing
46 Lower Green Road,Esher KT10 8HD

For more information on healing send a SAE to:

National Federation of Spiritual Healers
Old Manor, Farm Studio,
Church Street,
Sudbury on Thames
Middlesex, TW16 6RG
(0892 626080)

International Network of Esoteric Healing
15 Shakespeare Road, Worthing
W Sussex BN11 4AR
(01903 234125)

International Self-realisation healing Association
1 Hamlyn Road, Glastonbury
Somerset BA6 8HS
(01458 831353)

College of Healing
Runnings Park, Croft Bank
West Malvern, Worcs WR14 4DU
(01684 5664500)

NFSH Healer Referral Service
Tel: 0891 616080

For more information on counselling and Psychotherapy send a large SAE to:

British Association for Counselling (BAC)
1 Regents Place
Rugby, Warwickshire, CV21 2PJ
(01788 550899)

The National Council of Psychotherapist
Head Office
Hazelwood, Broadmead
Sway, Hants, SO41 6DH
(01590 683770)

UK Council for Phychotherapy (UKCP)
167-169 Great Portland Stsreet
London WIN 5FB
(020 7435 3002)

For more information on Reiki and a practitioners list send SAE to:

International Reiki Healers
10 Beach Houses, Royal Crescent,
Margate, Kent CT9 5AL
Tel 01843 231377

Reiki Association
Mel Jones, Cornbroook Bridge House,
Clee Hill, Ludlow, Shropshire SY8 3QQ
(01981 550829)

For more information on EMDR and a practitioner list send a SAE to:

EMDR Institute
P.O. Box 51010
Pacific Grove
USA
CA93950

EMDR UK
Tel 020 8951 3420

For more information of Feng Shui and a practitioner list send a SAE to:

Feng Shui Network International
Kings Court, Pateley Bridge, N Yorks
(01423 712868)

Assocation for Professional Therapists
Katepwa House, Ashfield Park Avenue
Ross-on-Wye, Herfordshire HR9 5AX
(01989 764905)

The Feng Shui Association
31 Woburn Place, Brighton, East Sussex BN1 9GA
(01273) 693844

For more information on herbal medicine and a list of practitioners send a SAE to:

General Council and resister of Consultant Herbalists
32 King Edwards Road,
Swansea SFA1 4LL
(01792 655886)

National Institute of Medical Herbalists
56 Longbrook Street, Exeter,
Devon EX4 6AH
(01392 426022)

United Register of Herbal Practitioners
PO Box 126, Crowborough TN7 4ZR
(01303 814816)

For more information on Hypnotherapy and a practitioner list send a SAE to:

British Hypnotherapy Association
67 Upper Berkeley Street, London WIH 7DH
(020 7723 4443)

The National Register of Hynotherapists and Psychotherapists
12 Cross Street, Nelson, Lancashire BB9 7EZ
(01282 699378)

For more information on Homeopathy and practitioner list send a large SAE to:
Homeopathy Research and Development Trust,
Hahnemann House, 32 Welbeck Street, London, W1M 7PG

Society of Homeopaths
2 Artisan Road, Northampton NN1 43HU
(01604 621400)

The Homeopathic Trust
15 Clerkenwell close, London EC1R OAA
(020 7566 7800)

The UK Homeopathic Medical Association
6 Livingstone Road, Gravesend, Kent DA12 5DZ
(01474 560336)

Homeopathy Research and Development Trust
Hahnemann House, 32 Welbeck Street, London, WIM 7PG

The European Therapy Studies Institute (ETSI)
Henry House, 189 Heene Road,
Worthing, West Sussex BNII 4NN

For more information about Iridology and practitioner list send SAE to:
Guild of Naturopathic Iridologists
94 Grosvenor Road, London SW1V 3LF
(020 7834 3579)

The Holistic Iridology Association
90 Tudor Drive, Morden, Surrey SM4 4PF

For more information on Nutritional Therapy and a list of practitioners send a cheque for £2.00 and a SAE to:

British Association of Nutritional Therapists
PO Box 17436, SW13 7WT

Institute of Optimum Nutrition
13 Blades Court, Deodar Road, London SW15 2NU
(020 8877 9993)

(Send a cheque for £1.00 and a SAE)
Society for the Promotion of Nutritional Therapy
PO Box 47 Heathfield, E Sussex TN21 8ZX
(01825 872921)

For more information about the Metamorphic technique send a SAE to:
The Metamorphic Association
67 Ritherdon Road
London SW17 8QE

For more information on Indian Head Massage and a list of practitioners send a SAE to:
London Centre of Indian Champissage
136 Holloway Road, London N7 8DD
(020 7609 3590)

For more information of kinesiology and a list of practitioners send a SAE to:
Association for Systemic Kinesiology
39 Browns Road, Surbiton
Surry, KT5 8ST

Kinesiology Federation
PO Box 17, Walmer Green
Knebworth S93 6UF
(01438 817998)

For further details about Light Therapy
The Hale Clinic
London Tel 0171 637 3377

For more information on Magnotherapy contract:
The Institute of Magnotherapy
Agrolaan 172, NL-4624 AN Bergen op Zoom, The Netherlands

For more information on massage and a list of practitioners send SAE to:
British Massage Therapy Council
78 Meadow Street, Preston, Lancashire PR1 1TS
(01772 881063)

Scottish Massage Therapists Association
70 Lochside Road, Denmore Park, Bridge on Don, Aberdeen B23 8QW
(01224 822960)

The Institute for Structural BodyWork
15 Water Lane, Kings Langley,Hertfordshire WD4 8HP
(0923) 268795

Manual Lymphatic Drainage
PO Box 149, Wallingford, Oxfordshire OX10 7LD

For more information and a list of Naturopathy practitioners send a cheque for £2.50 and a SAE to:
General Council and Register of Naturopaths
Goswell House, 2 Goswell Road, Street, Somerset BA16 OJG
(01458 840072)

For more information about nutrition send SAE to:
Women's Nutritional Advisory Service (PMT/Menopause)
P.O. Box 268 Hove.
W. Sussex
BN3 1RW

British Society of Nutritional And Environmental Medicine
PO Box Totton,
Southampton
S040 2ZA

Society for Promotion of Nutritional Therapy
P.O. Box 47
Heathfield
East Sussx
TN21 8ZX

British Society of Nutritional and Environmental Medicine.
PO box Totton, Southampton, SO40 2ZA

For more information on Osteopathy send a SAE to:
Osteopathic Information Service
Osteopathy House
176 Tower Bridge Road
London SE1 3LU
(020 7357)

For more information about reflexology and a list of practitioners send a large SAE to:
Association of Reflexologists
27Old Gloucester Street, London WC1N 3XX
(08705 673320)

The British Reflexology Council
Monks Orchard, Whitbourne, Worcester WR6 5RB
(01886 821207)

International Federation of Reflexologists
78 Edridge Road, Croydon, Surrey, CRO 1EF
(020 8667 9458)

For more information about Rolfing send a SAE to:
Rolf Institute
80 Clifton Hill, London, NW8 OJT
020 7328 9026

The International Rolf Institute
P.O. Box 1868, Boulder, CO 80306, USA.
(303) 449-5903

Or phone (020 7834 1493)

For more information about Rosen Method in the USA contact:
Rosen Institute
2325 Prince Street, Berkley, CA 94702, U.S.A
(415) 548-1205

For more information on shiatsu and a list of practitioners send a SAE to:
The Shiatsu Society
Barber House, Storeys Bar Road, Sengate, Peterborough PE1 5YS
(01733 75341)

The Shiatsu Society
31 Pullman Lane
Godalming
Surrey CU7 1XY

Shiatsu Society Secretary,
14 Oakdene Road.
Redhill, Surrey, RH1 6BT

Shiatsu Society
Barber House, Storeys Bar Road, Fengate, Peterborough
PE1 5YS

For more information about T'ai Chi and Martial arts and a list of registered practitioners send a SAE to:
UK T'ai Chi Association
142 Greenwich High Road, SW10 8NN
(020 8305 9571)

Martial Arts Commission
First Floor, Broadway House, 15/16 Deptford Broadway, London SE8 4PE
0181 691 8711

For information about Therapeutic Touch contact:
British Touch for Health Association
82a Highgate Road, London NW5 1PB
0171 267 0269

For more information about yoga and a list of practitioners send a SAE to:
Yoga Therapy Centre
Royal Homeopathic Hospital
60 Great Ormand Street, London WCIN 4HR
(020 7419 7195)

Wheel of Yoga
1 Hamilton Place, Boston Road, Sleaford, Lincs NG34 7ES
(01529 306851)

Yoga Health Foundation
Ickwell Bury, Ickwell Green, Northill
Biggleswade, Bedfordshire SG18 9EF
(076727 271)

Transcendental Meditation
Freepost
London SWIP 4YY
0800 269303

Other Useful Addresses

Research and Information in Complementary Medicine
60 Great Ormond Street, London WC14 3JF

Dr Helena Waters
Life Foundation School of Therapeutics
Maristow House. Dover Street, Bilston, W Midlands, WV14 6AL

For practitioner lists of most therapies send a SAE to:

The Federation of Holistic Therapists
38A Portsmouth Road, Woolston, Southampton, Hampshire SO199AD

The Guild of Complementary Practitioners
Liddell House, Liddell Close, Finchampsted, Berkshire, RG40 4NS

Council for Complementary and Alternative Medicine.
38 Mount Pleasant, London WCIX OAP

National Association for Premenstrual Syndrome
P.O. Box 72 Sevenoaks, Kent TN13 1XQ

Eating Disorders Association
Sackville Place, 44 Magdalen Street, Norwich, NR3 1JU

Relate - National Marriage Guidance
Herbert Grey College
Little Church Street
Rugby, CV21 3AP

Research into Ageing
Baird House. 15/17 St Cross Street
London EC1N 8UN

Migraine Action Association
178a High Road, Byfleet.
Surrey KT14 7ED
(01932 352468)

(Supplier of Melatonin and Light boxes, Full Spectrum Light and Natural Alarm Clocks)

SR-3 International
Tools For Energy, Balance and Health
25 Hainthrorpe Road, London SE27 OPL
(07000-822-496)

(Usefull address for Snoring and Sleep Apnoea)

British Snoring and Sleep Apnoea Association.
How Lane , Chipstead , Surrey, CR5 3LT
(01737 557997)

American Sleep Disorders Association
6301 Bandel Road, Suite 101, Rochester, MN 55901

IBS Network
c/o Centre for Human Nutrition
Northern General Hostital
Sheffield. S5 7AU
Run by IBS sufferers for IBS sufferers.

(Address for IBS Suffers)

IBS Network

St Johns House, Hither Green Hospital
Hither Green Lane, London SE13 6RU
(020 8698 4611)

(Usefull Address for Vitamins and Supplements)
Goldshield Professional Care
P.O. Box 789, Thornton Health, Surrey, CR7 7XT

(Addresses for Depression and Mental illness Depressives Associated)
P.O. Box 1022, London, SE1 7QB
(support and help from ex-depressives)
(020 7721 7672)

Granta House
15-19 Broadway, Stratford, London, E15 4BQ
(ring to find your nearest self-help group)
(020 8519 2122)

(For sleep problems and advise with beds)
The Sleep Council,
High Corn Mill, Chapel Hill, Skipton BD23 1NL
(01756 791089)

British Tinnitus Association
14/18 West Bar Green, Sheffield S1 2DA
(0114 279 6600)

(Children victims of abuse)
Childline
Free post 1111, London N1 OBR
(0800 1111)

(Cruse - Bereavement Care)
Cruse House, 126 Sheen Road, Richmond TW9 IUR
(Help line) 0181 331 7227

Eating Disorders Association
Sackville Place, 44 Magdalen Street, Norwich, NB3 1JU
(01603 621414) (adult helpline)
(01603 765050)(youth helpline)

Impotence Association
(020 8767 7791)

National Association for Premenstrual Syndrome
PO. Box 72, Sevenoaks, Kent, TN13 1XQ
(01732 741709)

Relate - National Marriage Guidance
Herbert Grey College, Little Church Street, Rugby CV21 3AP
(01788 573241)
For local Relate centres, look in telephone book under R

The British Astrological and Psychic Society
Bletchingley Road, Nutfield, Surrey RH1 4HW
(01293 542326)

Myalgic Encephalomyelitis Association
PO Box 8, Stanford le Hope, Essex SS17 8EX
(0375 642466)

National Osteoporosis Society
PO Box 10, Radstock, Bath BA3 3YA
(01761 471771)

Disabled Living Foundation
380-384 Harrow Road
London, W9 2HU
(0870 603 9177)

(for information about Restless Legs Syndrome)
Ekbom Support Group
2 The Green, Chedburgh, Bury St Edmunds, Suffolk IP29 4UE
(01284 850281)

(for information about Eczema)
National Eczema Society
163 Eversholt Street, London NW1 1BU
(020 7388 4097)

(for information about allergies.)
Action Against Allergy
P.O. Box 278, Twickenham TW1 4QQ
020 8892 2711

Appendix 2

Further Reading

(Coming off Prescription Pills)
Coming off Tranquillizers, Sleeping Pills and Anti-depressants, Shirley Trickett, Thorsons, 1998.

(Managing Pain)
Coping Successfully with Pain, Neville Shone, Sheldon Press, 1992.

(Tinnitus)
Tinnitus, Living with noises in your head, Michael O'Toole, Souvenir Press Ltd, 1995.

(Headaches and Migraines)
Headaches and Migraines, Dr J N Bau, Hodder and Stoughton, 1991.

(Diabetes)
Diabetes at your fingertips, Peter Sonksen, Charles Fox and Sue Jubb, Class Publishing Ltd, 1991

(Stress and Depression)
Which: Managing Stress, Mark Greener, Which Books, 1996
Geopathic Stress, How Earth ENergies Affect Out Lives, Jane Thurness-Read, Element, 1995.

(Menopause and Menstrual problems)
A Change for the Better, A womans guide through the menopause, Patricia Davies, Saffron Walken, The C.W. Davis Co Ltd, 1993.
Manstrual and Pre-menstrual Tension, Jan de Vries, Mainstread Publishing Co Ltd. 1992.

(M. E.)
M.E. and you, *A survivors guide to Post-viral fatigue syndrome*, Steve Wilkinson, Thorsons Publishing Group. 1988.

(I.B.S.)
Irritable Bowel Syndrome and Diverticulosis, Shirley Trickett, Thorsons, 1990.

(Reflexology)
The Reflexology handbook, A complete guide, Pauline wills, Element, 1998

(Reflexology and Colour Therapy)
Reflexology and Colour Therapy, Pauline Willis, Element, 1998.

(Aromatherapy)
The Directory of Essential Oils, Wanda Sellar, The C.W. Daniels Co Ltd, 1997.
Aromatherapy, Chrissie Wildwod, Bloomsbury, 1996.
Aromatherapy an A-Z, Patricia Davies, The C.W. Daniel Co Ltd, 1997.

(Aromatherpy and Ayurveda)
Ayurveda and Aromatherapy.
Dr Light Miller ND, and Dr Bryan Miller, DC, Lotus Press, 1995

(Colour and Crystal therapy)
Colour your life, Howard and Dorothy Sun, Judy Piatkus Ltd, 1992
Healing with Crystals and Gemstones, Daya Sarai Chocron, Samuel Weiser, inc, 1983.
Colour Therapy, The use of colour for health and healing, Pauline Wills, Elementy, 1995.

(Herbal Medicine)
Holistic Woman's Herbal, Kitty Campion, Bloomsbury, 1995
The Holistic Herbal, Mrs M Grieve, Tiger Books International, 1992.

(Nutrition and Food)
Your body's many cries for water, Dr F Batmanghelidj, Pulished by the Therapist Ltd, 1997
Complete Food Combining, all you need to know about the Hay diet, Peter and Donna Thomson, Bloomsbury Publishing, 1996
Your Healing Power, Jack Angelo, Piatkus, 1999.

280

Appendix 3

Ten Point Flexibility Plan

This daily programme of warming up exercises starts from your head and works down to your feet. Repeat each exercise ten or twelve times. Only work to your own stretching ability never over stretch your body, try to increase your flexibility slowly, day by day.

If you feel that some to the exercises are beyond you, do the ones you can manage and try again later to master the others. Walk a little bit each day and try to increase the time and distance bit by bit. As you get used to it, try to walk a little faster, too; it will also benefit your heart.

1. Drop you chin on to your chest and slowly roll your head from side to side.

2. Make circles with your shoulders by lifting them up towards your ears as far as they will go, pulling them backwards and then letting them drop down again repeat in the opposite direction.

3. Swing both arms in big circles, then change directions and repeat.

4. Rotate hands and wrist first one way then the other and stretch out your fingers and clench them.

5. Keeping your hips still, turn the upper half of your body from side to side. Do this fairly slowly and gently and don't try to increase the movement by swinging your arms.

6. Make big circles with your hips as if you were swinging a hula-hoop. Repeat in the opposite direction.

7. Bend your knees as far as they will comfortable go and press up again.

8. Hold on to something firmly and swing one leg backwards and forwards slowly, then swing the other leg.

9. Sitting stretch out your legs in front of you and hold.

10. Rotate each foot slowly round in one direction and then the other, stretch out and clench toes.

Appendix 4

Sleep Diary Guide Lines

Buy an A4 or A5 exercise book or page a day diary and record your sleep and your dreams in it every day.

You will find it very helpful to record some of the following information:

Day and Date

- The date and day

- Any out of the ordinary occurrences during the day or next i.e. meeting at work the following morning, argument with partner, illness, out of the ordinary travelling and moving house.

Times of going to bed and sleeping

- Time or going to bed

- Time approximately of going to sleep

- If waking during the night, time duration (did you get up and do something, or lie there for a while)

- If went back to sleep.

- Time when you wake up in morning

- Time that you get up in morning.

- Did you wake refreshed or tired?

- Did you nap during the day?

Food, drink and drug intake

- Foods eaten during day

- Foods eaten during evening and timing

- Tea coffee eaten during evening

- Alcohol intake and timing

- Smoking intake

- Prescribed drugs intake and timings

- Over the counter drugs and timings

- Illegal drugs intake and timing

Natural therapies tried

- Herbal medicines taken and timing

- Homeopathic remedies taken and timing

- Aromatherapy

- Massage

- Reflexology

- Or any other remedies or therapies

- Exercise taken

- What exercise

- How long

- What time

Dreams

- What you dreamed

- Description of dream

- How you're felt afterwards

- How much you remembered

Did you see any messages that relate to your life?

Bibliography

A-Z of the Human Body, Readers Digest Association Ltd. 1987.

Your body's many cries for water, Dr F. Batmanghelidj, Published by the Therapist Ltd. 1997.

The Secrets of Natural Health, Shyam Singha, Element, 1997.

The Insomnia Book, Dr Chris Idzikowski, Newleaf, 1999.

The Optimum Nutrition Bible, Patrick Holford, Piatkuk, 1997.

Irritable Bowel Syndrome and Diverticulosis, Shirley Trickett, Thorsons, 1990.

Complete Food Combining, All you need to know about the Hay diet, Peter and Donna Thomson, Bloomsbury Publishing, 1996.

Natural Prescriptions, Effective Treatments for over 100 Common Complaints, Dr Robert Gillerwith Kathy Matthews, Carol Southern Books, 1994.

Princicles of Shiatsu, Chris Jarmey, Thorsons. 1997.

Colour Therapy, The use of colour for health and healing, Pauline Wills, Element, 1993

Natural Remedies Common Ailments Cured, Gordon Sambidge, Piccadilly Press, 1995.

The Complete New Herbal, Richard Mabey, Elm Tree Books, 1988.

The Holistic Herbal, David Hoffmann, Finfhorn Press, 1983.

Coming off Tranquillizers, Sleeping Pills and Anti-depressants, Shirley Trickett, Thorsons, 1998.

Aromatherapy An A -Z, Patricia Davis, The C.W. Daniel Co Ltd, 1997.

Aromatherapy, Chrissie Wildwood, Bloomsbury, 1996.

Reflexology and Colour Therapy, Pauline Wills, Element, 1998.

The Reflexology Handbook, A complete guide, Larra Norman with Thomas Cowan, Piatkus, 1989.

The Alexander Technique Workbook, Richard Brennan, Element, 1997.

Acupressure, Michael Reed Cach, Piakus, 1997.

The Directory of Essential Oils, Wanda Sellar, The C.W. Daniel Co Ltd, 1997.

The Which? Guide to Complementary Medicine, Barbara Rowlands, Penguin Group, 1997.

Ayurveda and Aromatherapy, Dr Light Miller ND, and Dr Bryan Miller, DC, Lotus Press, 1995.

Healing with Crystals and Gemstones, Daya Sarai Chocron, Samuel Weiser, inc, 1983.

Which: Managing Stress, Mark Greener, Which Books, 1996.

A Change for the Better, A Woman's Guide through the Menopause, Patricia Davis, Saffron Walden, The C.W. Daniel Co Ltd, 1993.

The Herb Society's Complete Medicinal Herbal, Penelope Ody Minimh, Dorling Kindersley, 1993.

A Medern Herbal, Mrs M. Grieve, Tiger Books International,1992.

The Holistic Herbal, David Hoffmann, Findhorn Press, 1983.

Geopathic Stress, How Earth Energies Affect Our Lives, Jane Thurnell-Read, Element, 1995.

M.E. and you, A survivors guide to Post-Viral Fatigue Syndrome, Steve Wilkinson, Thorsons Publishing Group, 1988.

Colour Your Life, Howard and Dorothy Sun, Judy Piatkus Ltd, 1992

Reflexology and Colour Therapy, Pauline Wills, Element, 1998.

Menstsrual and Pre-Menstrual Tension, Jan de Vries, Mainstream Publishing Co ltd, 1992.

Holistic Woman's Herbal, Kitty Campion, Bloomsbury, 1995.

Tinnitus, Living with noises in Your Head, Michael O'Toole, Souvenir Press Ltd, 1995.

Coping Successfully with Pain, Neville Shone, Sheldon Press, 1992.

Diabetes at your Fingertips, Peter Sonksen, Charles Fox and Sue Jubb, Class publishing Ltd. 1991.

Headaches and Migraines, Dr J N Blau, Hodder and Stoughton, 1991.

Crown Chakra

Brow Chakra

Throat Chakra

(Thymus Chakra)

Heart Chakra

Solar Plexus Chakra

Sacral Chakra

Base Chakra

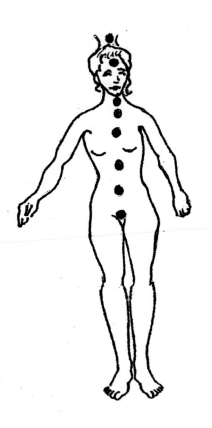

Appendix 5

The Chakras

There are seven or eight major centres within each level of the aura, which absorb colour vibrations and circulate them around the complete system. These are the centers of power, known as the 'Chakras' (from the Sanskrit word meaning Wheel of Fire), and they originated with the philosophy of the ancient yoga systems of India. The major chakras are listed below along with their associated locations, forces, sense organs and colours.

These centres are:
• The crown centre is located out of the body above the head or on top of the head, this is white or magenta, and is sometimes said to be related to upper brain to a higher state of consciousness, love and compassion are controlled here.

• The third eye or brow centre related to the nervous system and lower brain, when this centre is functioning properly it will aid sleep; this is our thinking centre, colour violet.

• The throat at the base of neck, related to the thyroid gland and breathing, speech and verbal communication are controlled here, colour blue.

• (The thymus chakra, situated between the heart chakra and the thyroid chakra, this position is not always recognized because as we grow older it diminishes; this area deals with growth and recovery, colour turquoise.)

• The heart related to the heart, thymus, blood and circulatory system, concerns harmony, balance and sharing with others, colour green.

• The solar plexus below the shoulder blades, related to the pancreas, stomach or naval, vitality and energy in the body generally, colour yellow.

• The sacral in the sacrum, lower part of the lumber spine, related to the adrenal gland and spleen, appetite and emotional expression are affected here, colour orange.

• And the basal located at the base of the spine, related to the spinal column and gonads; traditionally this chakra is associated with the seat of our life force energy and positive feelings, passion and friendship, colour red.

However, other authors sometimes use different names and locations, and these definitions are only intended as a guide.

The Chakras form part of the auric body including the physical body, and they are all constantly moving, continuously absorbing specific currents of energy. A free flow of this energy is vital to the health and well being of a person. All the chakras inter-connect with one another, and are joined within the body at intervals along the spine. Each of the seven (or eight including the thymus) chakras corresponds with a particular colour frequency, and with a particular gland or part of the human body. The chakras work to attract a dominant energy vibration, which can help to restore health and to maintain health in cases where disorder has caused blockage or resistance. In a healthy body, the chakras absorb and distribute energy evenly, in an unhealthy state; toxins may begin to collect which can eventually cause actual physical, emotional and mental problems if the charkas are out of balance. The natural rhythms of the body are out, thus the sleep cycles will be out of balance.

Spiritual Balance

Essential oils can be used to help balance each individual chakra and once put in balance, will allow you more control over your body, your sleep cycle and the ability to balance energy and transform your life.

• Crown Chakra, (Lavender, frankincense and rosewood) for spirituality and enlightenment.

• Third Eye, (Hyacinth, violet and rose geranium) for bringing intuition and wisdom.

• Throat, (chamomile and myrrh) for communication, and to assist self-expression and creativity.

• (Thymus), (basil, eucalyptus and thyme) for revival, to calm and restore.

• Heart, (bergamot, melissa and rose) for helping love and relationships.

• Solar Plexus, (vetiver, ylang ylang and bergamot) to promote personal power and self will.

• Sacral, (jasmin, rose and sandalwood) for emotional balance and sexuality.

• Root (Basal), (cedarwood, myrrh, patchouli) for survival and physical needs.

Chakra Meditation

First do the relaxation breathing exercise.

Then imagine you are lying on a beautiful white sandy beach at the edge of a coral reef. The warmth of the sun relaxes you as your body molds into the sand and warm clear turquoise blue water laps at your toes. With each breath the tension eases as your muscles start to relax, you are safe, warm and comfortable. Now, as you breathe in, take your attention to your feet and imagine the warm, clear blue water flowing in, gently massaging them before draining away at the base of the heel. As the water drains into the sand it removes any pain or tension, leaving your feet feeling warm and very relaxed. Continue this process throughout the whole of the body, legs, hips, and base of the spine, stomach, chest, arms, hands, shoulders, neck, face and head.

Enjoy this sense of well-being and imagine again the warmth of the sun as you breathe slowly, in and out, in via the mouth and out via the nose.

Now, take your attention back to the base of the spine and as you breathe deeply into this area, imagine a shoal of red fish swim in, filling the whole area with a bright red energy. Now breathe that red energy upwards into your abdomen as a shoal of yellow fish swim in, and as they mingle with the red fish, the area turns a bright orange. Now as the red fish swim away bring your breath and attention to your solar plexus, leaving the area bathed in yellow light. Next, as you breathe into the area around your heart, all the fish swim away and fronds of green ferns fill the area, gently massaging the heart. Moving on into the space around the throat and neck the fronds float away leaving only the bright clear blue turquoise water. Now, as your attention comes into the head and rests at the point in the middle of your forehead you swim through a cool indigo pool of water, and deep blue energy fills the area. As your attention comes, finally, to the top of your head you break the surface and brilliant white light streams through your body removing any last tension, thus renewing your chakras, leaving you very relaxed and with a renewed sense of well-being.

(This beautiful image was devised by Helen Bee who does some workshops and relaxation exercise classes)

Aura

All matter is constantly exchanging vibrations of different wavelengths. These vibrations affect us even though they may not be visible to the eye, and we may not be aware of their existence. The part of the electromagnetic spectrum, which surrounds us and penetrates us, represents our 'aura'.

Each of us can create our own magnetic atmosphere, and it will reveal our nature, temperament, character and state of well-being at that precise moment. The aura is like an antenna, capable of receiving information and sending out messages. Each of us can learn to become more sensitive to pick up vibrations from auras.

The aura or etheric body has been known to many cultures since ancient times, the seers of India and China have often described it, making diagrams to illustrate their finding. Other aboriginal cultures such as the Native American, Polynesian and Australian were aware of the etheric energy system and this has been depicted in their art, music and oral traditions.

In spite of this evidence, the presence of an energy field around living things was often written off by science because it could not be detected by modern technology. Then, in the 1890s a Polish nobleman, Yakub Yodko-Narkevitch, found a new form of photography which used a high voltage, high frequency electric charge instead of light this enabled him to photograph the energy field or aura that surrounds all living beings.

Studies in other parts of the world went on to discover that the light and colour given out varied according to the mood, or living force present. For example, a leaf plucked straight from a tree showed an energy field with grew smaller as the leaf dried out and died.

Semyon Kirian discovered Kirlian photography accidentally in 1939, a charge was passed across a film on which certain samples had been placed and strange light patterns were found to occur around them. Kirlian photography has shown that there seems to be an invisible shape or energy blueprint at the bio-energy level from which every living thing develops. Photographs of feet with missing toes show the energy figure as complete; this could also explain why some amputees still feel pain or sensation in missing limbs.

Index

FREE DETAILED
CATALOGUE

Capall Bann is owned and run by people actively involved in many of the areas in which we publish. A detailed illustrated catalogue is available on request, SAE or International Postal Coupon appreciated. **Titles can be ordered direct from Capall Bann, post free in the UK** (cheque or PO with order) or from good bookshops and specialist outlets.

Angels and Goddesses - Celtic Christianity & Paganism, M. Howard
Arthur - The Legend Unveiled, C Johnson & E Lung
Astrology The Inner Eye - A Guide in Everyday Language, E Smith
Auguries and Omens - The Magical Lore of Birds, Yvonne Aburrow
Asyniur - Womens Mysteries in the Northern Tradition, S McGrath
Beginnings - Geomancy, Builder's Rites & Electional Astrology, Nigel Pennick
Between Earth and Sky, Julia Day
Book of the Veil , Peter Paddon
Caer Sidhe - Celtic Astrology and Astronomy, Michael Bayley
Call of the Horned Piper, Nigel Jackson
Cat's Company, Ann Walker
Celtic Faery Shamanism, Catrin James
Celtic Faery Shamanism - The Wisdom of the Otherworld, Catrin James
Celtic Lore & Druidic Ritual, Rhiannon Ryall
Celtic Sacrifice - Pre Christian Ritual & Religion, Marion Pearce
Celtic Saints and the Glastonbury Zodiac, Mary Caine
Circle and the Square, Jack Gale
Compleat Vampyre - The Vampyre Shaman, Nigel Jackson
Creating Form From Mist - The Wisdom of Women in Celtic Myth, L. Sinclair-Wood
Crystal Clear - A Guide to Quartz Crystal, Jennifer Dent
Crystal Doorways, Simon & Sue Lilly
Crossing the Borderlines - Guising, Masking & Ritual Animal Disguise, Nigel Pennick
Dragons of the West, Nigel Pennick
Earth Dance - A Year of Pagan Rituals, Jan Brodie
Earth Harmony - Places of Power, Holiness & Healing, Nigel Pennick
Earth Magic, Margaret McArthur
Eildon Tree (The) Romany Language & Lore, Michael Hoadley
Enchanted Forest - The Magical Lore of Trees, Yvonne Aburrow
Eternal Priestess, Sage Weston
Eternally Yours Faithfully, Roy Radford & Evelyn Gregory
Everything You Always Wanted To Know About Your Body, But So Far
        Nobody's Been Able To Tell You, Chris Thomas & D Baker

Face of the Deep - Healing Body & Soul, Penny Allen
Fairies in the Irish Tradition, Molly Gowen
Familiars - Animal Powers of Britain, Anna Franklin
Forest Paths - Tree Divination, Brian Harrison, Ill. S. Rouse
From Past to Future Life, Dr Roger Webber
Gardening For Wildlife Ron Wilson
God Year, The, Nigel Pennick & Helen Field
Goddess Year, The, Nigel Pennick & Helen Field
Goddesses, Guardians & Groves, Jack Gale
Handbook For Pagan Healers, Liz Joan
Handbook of Fairies, Ronan Coghlan
Healing Book, The, Chris Thomas and Diane Baker
Healing Homes, Jennifer Dent
Healing Journeys, Paul Williamson
Healing Stones, Sue Philips
Herb Craft - Shamanic & Ritual Use of Herbs, Lavender & Franklin
In Search of Herne the Hunter, Eric Fitch
Inner Mysteries of the Goths, Nigel Pennick
Inner Space Workbook - Develop Thru Tarot, C Summers & J Vayne
Intuitive Journey, Ann Walker Isis - African Queen, Akkadia Ford
Journey Home, The, Chris Thomas
Language of the Psycards, Berenice
Legend of Robin Hood, The, Richard Rutherford-Moore
Lid Off the Cauldron, Patricia Crowther
Light From the Shadows - Modern Traditional Witchcraft, Gwyn
Lore of the Sacred Horse, Marion Davies
Lost Lands & Sunken Cities (2nd ed.), Nigel Pennick
Magic of Herbs - A Complete Home Herbal, Rhiannon Ryall
Magical Guardians - Exploring the Spirit and Nature of Trees, Philip Heselton
Magical History of the Horse, Janet Farrar & Virginia Russell
Magical Lore of Animals, Yvonne Aburrow
Magical Lore of Cats, Marion Davies
Magical Lore of Herbs, Marion Davies
Magick Without Peers, Ariadne Rainbird & David Rankine
Masks of Misrule - Horned God & His Cult in Europe, Nigel Jackson
Medicine For The Coming Age, Lisa Sand MD
Menopausal Woman on the Run, Jaki da Costa
Mirrors of Magic - Evoking the Spirit of the Dewponds, P Heselton
Moon Mysteries, Jan Brodie
Mysteries of the Runes, Michael Howard
Mystic Life of Animals, Ann Walker
New Celtic Oracle The, Nigel Pennick & Nigel Jackson
Oracle of Geomancy, Nigel Pennick
Pagan Feasts - Seasonal Food for the 8 Festivals, Franklin & Phillips
Patchwork of Magic - Living in a Pagan World, Julia Day
Pathworking - A Practical Book of Guided Meditations, Pete Jennings

Personal Power, Anna Franklin
Pillars of Tubal Cain, Nigel Jackson
Practical Divining, Richard Foord
Practical Meditation, Steve Hounsome
Practical Spirituality, Steve Hounsome
Psychic Self Defence - Real Solutions, Jan Brodie
Real Fairies, David Tame
Reality - How It Works & Why It Mostly Doesn't, Rik Dent
Romany Tapestry, Michael Houghton
Sacred Animals, Gordon MacLellan
Sacred Celtic Animals, Marion Davies, Ill. Simon Rouse
Sacred Dorset - On the Path of the Dragon, Peter Knight
Sacred Grove - The Mysteries of the Forest, Yvonne Aburrow
Sacred Geometry, Nigel Pennick
Sacred Nature, Ancient Wisdom & Modern Meanings, A Cooper
Sacred Ring - Pagan Origins of British Folk Festivals, M. Howard
Seasonal Magic - Diary of a Village Witch, Paddy Slade
Secret Places of the Goddess, Philip Heselton
Secret Signs & Sigils, Nigel Pennick
Self Enlightenment, Mayan O'Brien
Spirits of the Earth series, Jaq D Hawkins
Stony Gaze, Investigating Celtic Heads John Billingsley
Stumbling Through the Undergrowth , Mark Kirwan-Heyhoe
Symbols of Ancient Gods, Rhiannon Ryall
Talking to the Earth, Gordon MacLellan
Taming the Wolf - Full Moon Meditations, Steve Hounsome
The Other Kingdoms Speak, Helena Hawley
Tree: Essence of Healing, Simon & Sue Lilly
Understanding Chaos Magic, Jaq D Hawkins
Water Witches, Tony Steele
Way of the Magus, Michael Howard
West Country Wicca, Rhiannon Ryall
Wildwitch - The Craft of the Natural Psychic, Poppy Palin
Wondrous Land - The Faery Faith of Ireland by Dr Kay Mullin
Working With the Merlin, Geoff Hughes
Your Talking Pet, Ann Walker

FREE detailed catalogue and FREE 'Inspiration' magazine

Contact: Capall Bann Publishing, Auton Farm, Milverton, Somerset, TA4 1NE